MW01357710

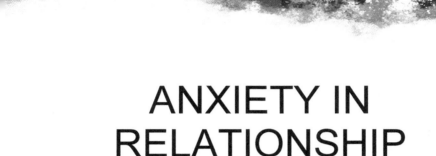

ANXIETY IN RELATIONSHIP

HOW TO GET RID OF ANXIETY
AND KEEP A LONG-TERM
RELATIONSHIP IN LOVE.
LEARN HOW TO OVERCOME
NEGATIVE THINKING,
JEALOUSLY AND INSECURITY
EASILY. A PRACTICAL HELP
FOR COUPLES

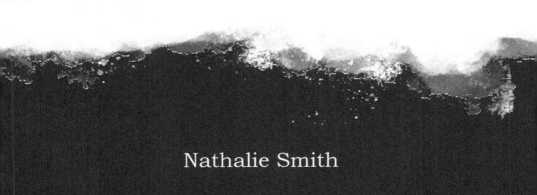

Nathalie Smith

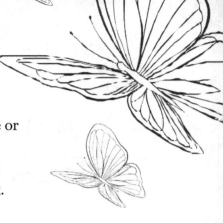

TABLE OF CONTENTS

Introduction

We have all established relationships throughout our lives. We began making connections with others at an early age within the family unit with our parents and siblings. As we grew up, we developed other relationships of friendship and love. Although every relationship is different, during the research process for this book, we had the opportunity to study its dynamics and noticed that there is one common factor that robs every one's happiness: **anxiety**.

Anxiety is also a universal, emotional feeling that is part of all activities in our lives. In itself, is not a negative feeling, as its natural function is to alert us to possible threats so that we can accurately assess them and respond effectively. When anxiety becomes persistent and is caused by significant emotional distress, it can cause disorders such as fear, phobia, and obsession. In these situations, anxiety can have profoundly distressing effects on our lives, our physique, and our mental health.

Research from the *Anxiety and Depression Association of America* says that about 40 million Americans, 18% of the population, have an anxiety disorder[1]. A joint study by the *Center for Emotional Intelligence and the Child Study Center* at Yale and Leipzig Universities, reported in *The New York Times*, pointed out that 1 in

---

[1] ANXIETY & DEPRESSION ASSOCIATION OF AMERICA, adaa.org.

7

5 workers, about 20% of the total, are at serious risk of burnout. Among the biggest causes of anxiety disorder are unemployment, health, and finances.

Our book will help you recognize the problems that cause anxiety in your life and your love relationship. You may have wondered: what's wrong with me? Why am I so jealous? Why don't my relationships last long? Will I ever be happy in a relationship?

You are not the only one who has asked yourself these questions. Everyone wants a successful, stable, and honest relationship with a partner with whom they can share their life. At the same time, however, people are hesitant to show their true selves to their partners and leave themselves vulnerable because they fear their fears will destroy their relationship. Hiding these personality traits does not help build a solid relationship. On the contrary, over time, it crumbles the relationship.

Thanks to this book you will be able to:

- **Identify the warning signs** of anxiety in yourself;

- Acquire **methods to manage them** when they hurt our emotions;

- **Recognize** if others around us such as friends, family, and colleagues are suffering from or at risk of distressing anxiety due to life events and circumstances;

- **Acquire practical communication skills**;

- **Address problems** in your relationship;

- **Overcome** anger, jealousy, negative thinking, insecure attachments, fear, and emotional problems;

- **Manage your anxiety** and the stress that comes with it.

Once you begin to better understand anxiety, you can do a lot to reduce the pressure and learn to feel the full spectrum of emotions.

If you're looking for comfort, reassurance, and support but don't know where to start, this book is for you! Happy reading.

Chapter 1: Anxiety or Anxiety Disorder?

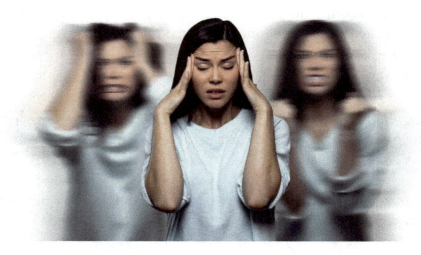

The word "*anxiety*" makes us think of a negative emotional state. In reality, anxiety is critical to our survival. If we perceive danger or believe that something dangerous will happen, our brain immediately sends a message to the rest of the body and the body responds by releasing dopamine. The increase in dopamine makes us feel strong and alert and prepares us *to strike (fight) or flee for survival (escape).*

Another way anxiety comes to our aid is when we have a job to finish on a deadline, need to prepare for an exam, pay bills, or complete any other task throughout the day.

The increase in adrenaline, however, can have negative side effects that differ from subject to subject, such as nervousness, apprehension, insomnia, apnea, sensitivity to crying, palpitations, weakness and stomach cramps, swollen belly, a lump in the throat, shortness of breath, fatigue, variable mood cycles, continuous gestures, unwarranted phobias, panic attacks and finally obsessive-compulsive disorders. Despite this, anxiety attacks are not permanent and usually last from a few minutes to a few hours.

Anxiety can affect your physique: it can raise (or lower) your blood pressure, raise your white blood cells, and suddenly alter your blood sugar levels due to the action of adrenaline on your liver. It can even alter your cardiogram. Dr. Charles Mayo said: *"Anxiety affects the circulation, the heart, the glands, the whole nervous system".* [2]

Although anxiety can be unpleasant, it can get you through difficult situations quickly and help you do a better job. Ordinary anxiety is a feeling that recurs but does not interfere with your daily life. In an anxious condition, the feeling of **fear** can be with you at all times. This feeling is intense and often paralyzing and increases anxiety levels. Fear increases anticipation, desires, neurological body function and activates other behavioral tendencies. Since these two emotional states are very similar and are one consequence of the other, how can we distinguish between anxiety and fear?

Fear often has an immediate response that causes classic *fight-or-flight* reflexes. An unconscious fear reaction is faster than conscious thought and allows the body to release adrenaline

---

[2] STEINCROHN P. –LaFia D., *How to Master Your Nerves*, 1970, 14.

spikes, which can diminish until the anticipated or actual danger passes. This can be an ambiguous and uncomfortable feeling in anticipation of other misfortunes that are not clearly described. Unlike fears, anxiety is distinguished as a "warning response to real or extreme danger (real or perceived)" as "a potential state of mind in the final planning of potential negative events.

Generally, in the course of our days, we all face situations that cause feelings of anxiety. Anxiety encompasses mood states such as discomfort, agitation, or worry. In 2008 the journalist Harriet Grenn in an article in *The Guardian* said that *"we are entering a new era of anxiety"*[3]; of the same opinion was Patrick O'Connor, who in 2014 in *The Wall Street Journal* wrote that *"record levels of anxiety are being recorded among Americans"*[4]. Since we live in a world full of uncertainties, a few episodes of anxiety can happen to anyone. Each of us reacts differently when faced with a state of worry. Since anxiety is generated by a combination of factors such as genetics, one's lived history, stress, and past trauma, this implies that it is subjective. The same situation may create a mild state of worry in one person but create a panic attack in another.

Anxiety or anxiety disorder can therefore be a complex problem. Among its various causes are illness, old age, job loss, and concern for the well-being of the family. Anxiety, if properly motivated, is a transitory feeling with a positive effect. It becomes a problem when anxious episodes occur without real justification due to incomprehensible and non-affective reasons.

---

[3] THE GUARDIAN, Sun. 17 Aug. 2008.
[4] THE WALL STREET JOURNAL, *Poll Finds Widespread Economic Anxiety*, 5 Aug. 2014.

In these cases, overreactions can occur and anxiety becomes pathological or negative. If the cognitive, physical, and behavioral symptoms of anxiety are persistent and severe, and the concerns in an individual's life are so distressing to the point of negatively affecting the person's ability to work or learn, socialize, and conduct daily activities, it can go beyond healthy limits and become a full-blown disorder. When suffering from serious anxiety disorders, it would be wise to consult a specialist.

In most cases, pathological anxiety is accompanied by:

- **Panic attacks**: acute crises characterized by fear, palpitations, and disordered behavior. Most people have physical complaints, such as heart palpitations, swelling, anxiety, pain, heavy and fast breathing, dizziness, fainting, indigestion, stomach upset, nausea, and diarrhea. These circumstances prevent the person suffering from anxiety from relaxing and achieving normal sleep patterns and traps them in repetitive patterns of thought hindering normal lifestyle;

- **Phobias:** attitudes of real but not objective fear of contextual situations;

- **Obsessive-compulsive disorders**: characterized by recurring thoughts, images, or impulses. These trigger anxiety/disgust and "force" the person to perform repetitive material or mental actions to calm themselves.

In the case of **"chronic anxiety"**, it is necessary to intervene with long-term drug therapy, hypnotic-sedative medications, and possibly psychotherapy.

The American Psychological Association, or APA, referring to people with an anxiety disorder, says *"they have persistent intrusive thoughts or problems"*[5]. As soon as stress and anxiety reach the stage of an illness, it can hinder daily function. This kind of anxiety can cause you to stop doing things you appreciate. It may prevent you from entering an elevator, crossing the street, or even leaving the house in extreme cases. If neglected, anxiety will undoubtedly continue to worsen. Anxiety problems are one of the most common types of mental illness and can affect any person at any age. But what are the differences between an emotional state of anxiety and an anxiety disorder?

We briefly reviewed what anxiety is, the symptoms of an anxious state, the difference between anxiety and fear, and under what circumstances this intense emotion becomes a danger to our physical and mental health. Anxiety disorders are many and vary based on situations experienced in the past. Some of these disorders that affect our relationships with others are:

- Social anxiety and avoidant anxiety personality disorder (AvDP);

- Agoraphobia;

---

[5] AMERICAN PSYCHOLOGICAL ASSOCIATION, apa.org.

- Generalized Anxiety Disorder (GAD);

- Panic disorder (PD);

- Obsessive-compulsive disorder (OCD);

- Post-traumatic stress disorder (PTSD).

Let's analyze their main characteristics, triggers, and possible remedies.

Social Anxiety

Social anxiety is a type of anxiety disorder that arises from the *fear of being humiliated or rejected by other people.* The main characteristic of social phobia is the fear of acting in an embarrassing or humiliating way in front of other people, and therefore receiving negative judgments. The person suffering from it feels that those around him or she will scrutinize him or her. For this reason, the sufferer *avoids social events and gatherings* such as parties, dinners, or social gatherings. Sometimes it can create social anxiety to expose a relationship or even just sign in, make a phone call, eat or just walk into a room where there are people already sitting, or talk to one's friend. People with social phobia are afraid of appearing anxious and showing the "signs" of it, i.e., they are afraid of turning red in the face, shaking, stuttering, sweating, having a heartbeat, or remaining silent without being able to talk to others and without having the "ready" line.

Social anxiety can negatively affect an individual's relationships with loved ones. Sufferers can create a gap between themselves and their families.

If left untreated, social phobia tends to remain stable and chronic and can often give rise to other disorders such as depression. To overcome this disorder, it is crucial to discuss the symptoms of anxiety with loved ones and take action on time so that relationships and social life can be restored. It is important not to confuse social anxiety with shyness!

There are usually two types of Social Phobia:

- **Simple:** when the person experiences social anxiety in only one or a few types of situations (e.g., is unable to speak in public, but has no problem in other social situations such as attending a party or talking to a stranger);

- **Generalized:** when the person fears all social situations. In more severe and pervasive forms, the diagnosis of Avoidant Personality Disorder tends to be preferred.

Avoidant Personality Disorder or AvPD also called **anxious (avoidant) personality disorder**, is a personality disorder characterized by a penetrating behavior pattern of social inhibition, feelings of inadequacy, extreme sensitivity to negative evaluations of oneself, and a tendency to avoid social interactions.

People with an avoidant personality disorder often consider themselves socially inept or unattractive on a personal level and avoid social interactions for fear of being ridiculed, humiliated, or the object of dislike. Despite difficulties and strong inhibitions, **those with this disorder want to have social relationships.**

The avoidant personality disorder is diagnosed in early adulthood, but symptoms usually exist from childhood. Clinicians tend not to make a diagnosis at too young an age, as these characteristics may be normal for the age.

Speaking of the causes of anxiety, we have seen that they depend on numerous factors such as genetics and our history.

Also concerning avoidant personality disorder, the causes are to be found in emotional neglect, particularly rejection by one or both parents or perceived rejection by the peer group. People with this type of disorder are worried about their deficits and form relationships with others only if they believe they will not be rejected. The loss and rejection are so painful that these people will choose to remain alone rather than risk trying to relate to others. This anxiety disorder in the long run tends to cause stress, depression, and anxiety.

Treatment of avoidant personality disorder can make use of various techniques, such as social skills training, cognitive therapy, exposure treatment to gradually increase social contact, group therapy to practice social skills, and sometimes drug therapy.

Agoraphobia

The term **agoraphobia** comes from the Greek word *"Agora"* meaning square; in fact, the earliest uses of the word in psychology and psychiatry were for people who were afraid to go to crowded places.

Those suffering from agoraphobia fear situations in which it is difficult to escape or receive help; consequently, they avoid such places to control the anxiety related to the foreshadowing of a new panic crisis.

Situations most frequently avoided by those who exhibit symptoms of agoraphobia include: going out alone or staying home alone, driving or traveling by car, attending crowded places such as markets or concerts, taking the bus or airplane, being on a bridge, or in an elevator.

An individual suffers from agoraphobia when, to avoid any situation that could trigger a panic attack, they restrict themselves from performing daily activities by staying indoors for weeks or months, impairing daily activities and social-work functioning. Psychotherapy is essential for the treatment of agoraphobia.

Generalized Anxiety Disorder (GAD)

Generalized Anxiety Disorder (GAD) is a type of anxiety disorder in which a person endures a constant state of anxiety, often concerning small things.

It is characterized by apprehensive anticipation with pessimistic anticipation of negative or catastrophic events of any kind or nature. Sometimes it occurs even without apparent problems or stressors.

People who suffer from this anxiety disorder have difficulty sleeping and relaxing the mind.

In addition to having an excessive and uncontrollable worry about any circumstance, sufferers have common symptoms such as shortness of breath, headaches, muscle aches, nausea, tremor, sweating, irritability, dizziness, flushing, heartbeat, extrasystoles, nausea, diarrhea, dry mouth, a lump in the throat, musculoskeletal disorders, such as tension (especially in the neck and neck), tics, tremors, fatigability. The muscular tension typical of this disease can also express itself with diffuse Algic manifestations or headaches.

Subjects suffering from generalized anxiety disorder are often irritable, unable to relax, and even to maintain concentration, are described as often restless, distracted, and impatient. They frequently suffer from insomnia and brood over the possibility of impending misfortune for themselves and others.

This disorder occurs in any age group. Children with generalized anxiety disorder tend to worry too much about their performance, and over time, the core of the worry may shift from one object to another. The disorder (which tends to be chronic and long-lasting) can easily be accompanied by depression and lead to abuse of alcohol, caffeine, stimulants, and other substances.

To treat generalized anxiety disorder, psychotherapy is necessary.

The most effective psycho-therapies are cognitive-behavioral and address generalized anxiety in different ways:

- By separately addressing the various situations in which anxiety occurs through behavioral and cognitive restructuring techniques;

- By using relaxation techniques to interrupt the process of self-feeding anxiety and lower the general state of tension;

- Choosing interventions aimed at enhancing assertive skills.

Panic Disorder (PD)

Panic Disorder (PD) is a severe type of anxiety disorder that causes excessive and unexpected terror and keeps the individual in a state of near-constant fear. **Panic attacks** (also called panic crises) are episodes of *sudden, intense fear* or rapid escalation of normally present anxiety. They are accompanied by somatic and cognitive symptoms such as palpitations, sudden sweating, trembling, choking sensation, chest pain, nausea, dizziness, GAD, headache, muscle pain, and increased heart rate, fear of dying or going crazy, chills, or hot flashes.

Those who have experienced panic attacks describe them as a terrible experience, often sudden and unexpected, at least the first time.

The fear of a new attack immediately becomes strong and dominant. Although it is a single episode, it tends to easily lead to a real panic disorder, more for *"fear of fear"* than anything else.

A vicious circle is thus created that leads to *agoraphobia*, leading the person to avoid finding himself in places or situations from which it would be difficult or embarrassing to leave or in which help might not be available in case of an unexpected panic attack.

Therefore, with the fear of panic attacks, it becomes difficult and anxiety-inducing to leave the house alone, travel by train, bus, or car, to be in a crowd or a queue. Those suffering from panic disorder become slaves to panic, often forcing all family members to adapt accordingly, to never leave him alone and accompany him everywhere. The result is a sense of frustration that comes from being *"big and tall"* but at the same time dependent on others, which can lead to secondary depression.

Individuals with panic disorder exhibit characteristic concerns or interpretations about the implications or consequences of panic attacks. Concern about the next attack or its implications is often associated with the development of avoidance behaviors. This is referred to as **Panic Disorder with Agoraphobia.**

Attacks are usually more frequent during stressful periods. Some life events can act as precipitating factors, even if they do not necessarily cause a panic attack. Common precipitating life events include marriage or cohabitation, separation, loss or illness of a significant person, being a victim of some form of violence, and financial and work problems.

The first attacks usually occur in agoraphobic situations (such as driving alone or riding a bus in the city) and otherwise often in some stressful context.

Stressful events, hot and humid weather, and psychoactive drugs can trigger abnormal body sensations. These can be interpreted catastrophically, increasing the risk of developing panic attacks.

In the treatment of panic attacks with or without agoraphobia and anxiety disorders in general, the form of psychotherapy that scientific research has shown to be most effective is the *"cognitive-behavioral"*. This is relatively brief psychotherapy, usually, every week, in which the patient plays an active role in solving their problem. Together with the therapist, he or she focuses on learning ways of thinking and behaving that are more functional in treating panic attacks.

Obsessive-Compulsive Disorder (OCD)

Obsessive-compulsive disorder (OCD) is a condition in which an individual becomes unable to control his or her behavior and actions. Obsessive-compulsive disorder (OCD) can begin in childhood, adolescence, or early adulthood. In many cases, the first symptoms occur very early, in most cases before age 25.

Obsessive-compulsive disorder is characterized by recurring thoughts, images, or impulses. These trigger anxiety/disgust and "force" the person to perform repetitive material or mental actions to calm themselves.

Sometimes these two terms, obsessions and compulsions, are mistakenly used as synonyms. What is the difference between the two?

- **Obsessions** are intrusive, repetitive *thoughts*, images, or impulses that are perceived as uncontrollable by the person experiencing them. Such ideas are felt to be disturbing and usually judged as unfounded or excessive. Obsessions in *obsessive-compulsive disorder* activate unpleasant and very intense emotions, such as primarily anxiety, disgust, and guilt. As a result, sufferers feel the need to do everything possible to reassure themselves and manage their emotional distress.

- **Compulsions** typical of obsessive-compulsive disorder are also called ceremonial or ritualistic. They are *repetitive behaviors* (such as checking, washing/washing, ordering, etc.) or mental actions (praying, repeating formulas, counting) aimed at containing the emotional distress caused by the thoughts and impulses that characterize the obsessions described above. Compulsions easily become rigid rules of behavior and are decidedly excessive and sometimes bizarre.

Those who suffer from obsessive disorders may:

- Be exceedingly afraid of dirt, germs, and/or disgusting substances;

- Be terrified of inadvertently causing harm to themselves or others (of any nature: health, economic, emotional, etc.) through mistakes, carelessness, carelessness, carelessness;

- Fear that they may lose control of their impulses by becoming aggressive, perverse, self-damaging, blasphemous, etc.;

- Have persistent doubts about their feelings towards their partner or their sexual orientation, although they usually recognize that this is not justified;

- Feeling the need to perform actions and arrange objects always in the "right way," complete, "well done."

Some patients may have more than one type of disorder at the same time or at different times in their lives. The symptoms are obsessions and compulsions related to unlikely (or unrealistic) contagion or contamination. If the person comes into contact with one of the "contaminating" agents or otherwise feels a feeling of dirtiness, he/she enacts a series of compulsions (rituals) of washing, cleaning, sterilizing, or disinfecting. This is done to neutralize germs' action and reassure themselves about the possibility of infection or to get rid of the feeling of dirt and disgust.

People who suffer from this disorder tend to check and recheck; this is to make sure that they have done everything possible to prevent any possible catastrophe (sometimes to calm themselves about the obsessive doubt of having done something wrong and not remembering it).

Within this category are symptoms such as checking that you have closed the doors and windows of the house, the car doors, the gas and water taps, the garage door or the medicine cabinet, that you have turned off the electric stove or other appliances, the lights in every room of the house or the car headlights. Or that you didn't lose personal belongings by dropping them or unintentionally hit someone with your car.

The best treatment for obsessive disorders is cognitive-behavioral psychotherapy. It consists of two types of psychotherapy that complement each other:

- **Behavioral psychotherapy**: uses *exposure and response avoidance techniques*. Exposure to the anxiogenic stimulus is based on the fact that anxiety and disgust tend to decrease spontaneously after prolonged contact with the stimulus itself. For example, people with an obsession with germs may be asked to be in contact with objects "containing germs" (e.g., holding money) until the anxiety has disappeared. Repetition of exposure, which must be conducted in an extremely gradual and tolerable manner for the patient, allows the anxiety to diminish until it is completely gone.

It is necessary to combine the technique *of exposure* with the technique *of response prevention*, suspending or initially at least postponing, the usual ritualistic behaviors that follow the appearance of obsession;

- **Cognitive psychotherapy**: Cognitive psychotherapy aims to cure OCD through the modification of some automatic and dysfunctional thought processes. In particular, it acts on the excessive sense of responsibility, on the excessive importance attributed to thoughts, on the overestimation of the possibility of controlling one's thoughts, and on the overestimation of the danger of anxiety, which constitutes the main cognitive distortions of patients with OCD.

Post-Traumatic Stress Disorder (PTSD)

According to the DSM-IV-TR (APA, 2000), **Post-Traumatic Stress Disorder (PTSD)** develops following exposure to a stressful and traumatic event that the person experienced directly, or witnessed, and that involved death, or threats of death, or serious injury, or a threat to one's physical integrity or that of others.

Both adults and children may have to deal with traumatic events, and this can cause **post-traumatic stress disorder (PTSD).** A particular memory or flashback associated with the event can trigger a panic attack. People with post-traumatic stress disorder show increased irritability and emotional or physical outbursts when they experience a panic attack. Adults living with this PTSD tend to be depressed to abuse drugs.

Symptoms of PTSD can occur immediately after the trauma or months later.

Traumatic events experienced directly that can trigger this type of disorder can include all those situations in which the person felt in grave danger, such as military combat, violent personal assault, kidnapping, terrorist attack, torture, incarceration as a prisoner of war or in a concentration camp, natural or caused disasters, serious automobile accidents, rape, etc...

Events experienced as a witness include observing situations in which another person is seriously injured or witnessing another person's unnatural death due to violent assault, accident, war, or disaster, or being unexpectedly confronted with a dead body. Even just learning that a family member or close friend has been assaulted, had an accident, or died (especially if the death is sudden and unexpected) can trigger post-traumatic stress disorder.

The treatment of this type of anxiety disorder necessarily requires a cognitive-behavioral psychotherapeutic intervention, which facilitates the processing of trauma until the disappearance of anxiety symptoms.

How to Know If You or a Family Member Have Anxiety and What To Do

Anxiety makes no distinction between children, young people, or the elderly. People of all ages can suffer from anxiety disorders and there are many different causes and triggers for each.

For example:

- **In children and adolescents**: the most common anxiety-generating factors are pressure to do well in school, bullying by classmates or teachers, sibling rivalry, and upcoming exams. Many young children also face separation anxiety, which occurs when a child is permanently or temporarily separated from one or both parents.

- **In adults**: the causes of anxiety disorders tend to be work-related, traumatic events, the need to meet expectations, or the fear of failure.

- **In older people**: reasons for concern may relate to the onset of disability-inducing illness, perceptions of one's deterioration, poor financial security, or social isolation.

These situations put enormous **pressure on the person's psyche** and as a result, fear levels increase. Their mental health suffers and they begin to do poorly in school or at work. In addition to the psychological damage, their **physical health** will also take a hit. Stomach problems, irregular heartbeat, shortness of breath, nausea, sleep disturbances, and fatigue are physical manifestations of an anxiety disorder.

It has been shown that when talking about their problems, people with persistent anxiety have common thoughts and tend to ask the same questions such as:

- What if...?

- I can't cope.

- I will never be able to cope...

- This is too much for me! I'm going to fail!

- I am going crazy!

People with chronic anxiety have constant thoughts of worry and struggle to think about other things. However, people can have these thoughts and not necessarily have an anxiety disorder! Anxiety ranges from mild to severe and has different effects on each person. As mentioned earlier, anxiety is a completely natural behavior that all humans experience and is sometimes necessary to help identify potential danger. It only becomes dangerous and harmful when it crosses a line and becomes symptomatic. How can we tell if a person has an anxiety disorder?

Let's take a look at the difference between "everyday" anxiety and distressing distress to figure it out. Take, for example, a young person who prepares all afternoon because he has an exam at school the next day; he might be very irritable, think he can't present the material well, be afraid he'll forget something important, or think he won't hear the alarm clock ring in the morning.

Or think of a worker who has to finish a project quickly; they might be thinking about what could go wrong, be impatient, more irritable with their family, and maybe not be able to sleep at night.

Either way, **this could be "everyday" anxiety** or it could be a **sign of a different kind of anxiety**. How do we figure out which one it is?

At the beginning of the chapter, we saw what the symptoms of both anxiety and different anxiety disorders are. A practical way to tell if you or a family member suffers from anxiety is **to dwell on the duration and effects of the symptoms**, notice at what time they occur, and figure out if they always occur in the same way or if the severity of the symptoms increases whenever situations arise that generate high anxiety.

- If every time the same situation occurs, the symptoms are mild and always present in the same way and have the same duration, then it is likely that it is *"everyday anxiety"* and that is the way our body responds to that specific stressful situation.

- If in that same situation the symptoms always get worse or if you have anxiety disorder symptoms in other situations in life (sometimes for no apparent reason), it may not be an "everyday anxiety" disorder but a sign of an *anxiety disorder.*

By doing this, you will be able to determine if you are experiencing a situation that creates a *normal state of anxiety* with a rapid anxiety response or if you have a chronic *anxiety disorder*. If you believe that you or your family members have symptoms of chronic anxiety, you may want to seek professional help.

Chapter 2: What is Anxiety in Relationships and How Does It Start?

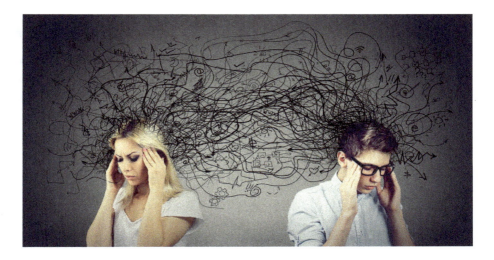

At least once in our lives we all want to find the right person to complete us and spend the rest of our lives with. However, although building a good relationship is one of the most enjoyable things in life, relying on another person can be a source of anxiety. Many people may experience feelings of anxiety and stress at the mere thought of finding themselves in a relationship. Even in the early stages of courtship, we may experience the effects of anxiety; for example, at the beginning of a relationship we may ask ourselves, *"Do I like this person?" "How serious is this relationship?" "Will it work?"* If we don't address these thoughts and allow room for anxiety, mistakenly thinking that "it will pass" will affect our relationship as it becomes more and more serious. At that point, we may be overwhelmed with thoughts like *"Do I like this person?" "Do I want to spend the rest of my life with him/her?" "Will he/she lose interest in me?"*

Ignoring signs of anxiety is never a good idea! Many people may be unaware that the way we relate to our partner is closely tied to the relationship we had with our mother.

Although a child relates to many figures that will be important throughout his or her life (father, grandparents, siblings, etc.), it is the **mother-child** attachment that will influence how he or she behaves in future romantic relationships. This is because the mother is the first person on whom the child is *completely* dependent in every aspect. The mother-child attachment creates a very deep imprint in how the child will see himself about others and expects to be accepted, loved, and understood in his uniqueness.

A **secure** mother-child attachment allows for the maturation of an adult who is more in touch with his or her own needs and able to talk about them, as he or she expects from the other a good commitment to understanding and then acceptance of who he or she is.

An **insecure attachment** (which can be avoidant, ambivalent, or disorganized) involves a whole series of fears and consequent behaviors, the more the relationship with the partner becomes intimate and important. What characterizes insecure attachment is precisely a strong level of anxiety related to the fear of abandonment. This anxiety is more evident if the attachment is ambivalent (or fearful) and less so if it is avoidant (or distancing). In both cases, anxiety causes a person who has grown up with this type of attachment to be constantly on the alert to avoid abandonment.

Anxiety:

- Forces one to maintain excessively high expectations toward oneself that clash with a perception of oneself as unworthy of love;

- Involves a strong and constant activation of alert systems, so you are hypervigilant about everything that happens, especially the behavior and thoughts of the partner;

- Encourages a distancing from one's true needs, since expressing them could result in a distancing or refusal to understand by the other.

How we relate to others varies from person to person and depends on how we express affection. Some look for a style of attachment in a partner that is compatible with their own, and those who are attracted to someone with a completely different style of attachment. In both cases, it is very important to keep an open mind and communicate with our partners. Lack of communication is one of the causes that generate anxiety in a relationship.

Let's first look at what the four attachment styles are. As we delve into them, figure out what **your** attachment style is by being honest with yourself. There is no such thing as a good and a bad attachment style, but there is the "best" one for you, the one that makes you feel safe, secure, and happy with your partner.

For example, if you find that you have an attachment style similar to the insecure one, but at the same time you feel that your partner understands you and is willing to accommodate you, then you will have found the "best" one for you.

Then try to figure out what your partner is as well. Take the time to reflect on your personality and past relationships, keeping in mind that people often exhibit characteristics of more than one attachment style. The ultimate goal of this research is to be able to have a happy, healthy, and lasting relationship.

There are four attachment styles and they are:

- Secure attachment;

- Insecure-ambivalent attachment;

- Insecure-avoidant attachment;

- Disorganized-disoriented attachment.

Let's analyze them one at a time.

Secure Attachment

As we have already said, the first years of life represent a period of fundamental importance for the child's healthy development and attachment system.

A type of attachment defined as **"secure"** provides the child with security and protection from vulnerability through closeness with the *caregiver* (the one who takes care of the child). Maternal sensitivity is crucial in this context.

Through a secure attachment style, the child learns functions that are fundamental to his or her development and is protected against the formation of violent behavior and antisocial cognitive and behavioral patterns. The specific attachment-related protective factors that reduce the risk of developing violent and aggressive behaviors in children are:

- the ability to regulate and modulate impulses and emotions;

- the development of pro-social values, empathy, and morality: secure attachment promotes pro-social values and behaviors that include empathy, compassion, kindness, and morality;

- the establishment of a strong, positive sense of self: children who have a secure foundation are more likely to be autonomous and independent throughout development. They explore the environment with little anxiety and greater skill, developing higher self-esteem, mastery skills, and self-differentiation. These children develop positive beliefs and expectations about themselves and interpersonal relationships (positive internal working model).

- Positive beliefs about self: 'I am good, wanted, competent and lovable';

- Positive beliefs about parents: 'they are responsive to my needs, sensitive and reliable';

- Positive beliefs about life: 'the world is safe, life is worth living;

- The ability to manage stress and adversity;

- The ability to create and maintain emotionally stable relationships: secure attachment implies an increased awareness of others' mental states, which not only produces a rapid development of morality but also protects the child from developing antisocial behavior.

In summary, we can say that: *the first years of life are a very important phase of development in which the child learns to trust, relational patterns, sense of self, and cognitive skills*. The secure attachment is the main protective factor against the formation of violent and antisocial behavior; thanks to a mother who can tune in to the needs of the child and provide presence and balanced rules, the child develops the skills necessary to regulate and modulate impulses and emotions, and to better manage stress and psychological trauma, develops pro-social and empathic behavior and is respectful of the rules. He can also learn to build a stable and solid sense of self, gradually become independent, explore the environment without anxiety, develop self-esteem, confidence in his abilities, and develop positive internal operating models about himself, others, and the world.

Adults with secure attachments are confident and comfortable with the full scope of their feelings. They are inclined to view their partners as trustworthy, supportive, and honest.

They know that their partner loves and understands them and, therefore, feel free to share anything with them. People with a secure attachment style offer the emotional support, loyalty, and implicit trust that their partners need.

When both you and your partner have aspects of the secure attachment style, you will find yourself in a lasting, stable, and healthy relationship.

Insecure-ambivalent Attachment

The **anxious-ambivalent attachment** style is characterized by the constant and compelling *need for reassurance and care* from the other. The child —and later the adult—who has this style of attachment in relationships**, is constantly worried and distressed** by the other's unpredictable behavior, to which he clings **fearing abandonment**. There are frequent outbursts of anger when the feeling of fear and insecurity prevails, excessive demand and/or claim of increasing attention, alternating with excessive surrender or submission to the other in relationships. Tends to develop over time an oppositional-provocative behavior, is unable to control impulses and emotions, is a liar, shows aggression and hyperactivity, and sometimes self-injurious behavior.

The attachment figures (*caregivers*) of children who have developed this style of attachment show **unpredictable and inconsistent** behavior towards the needs of care, protection, reassurance, and contact of the child.

At times they are welcoming and at other times refusing and devaluing; frequently inclined to aggressive behavior and not very emotionally involved with the child, they put him in the condition of not knowing what to expect in response to his requests and needs towards the reference figure, who is sometimes experienced as dangerous, and always as unpredictable. The child thus comes to develop two *"internal operating models"*:

- One characterized by the perception of self as lovable and worthy of love and the other as trustworthy and reliable;

- The other is characterized by the perception of oneself as unlovable and not worthy of love and the other as unavailable and/or dangerous.

These different internal models alternate in the individual's experience and perception, resulting in ambivalent and seemingly inconsistent behaviors toward the person with whom they relate.

People who exhibit this style of attachment often have difficulty dealing with problems in their social lives and professional lives. Because they need a lot of reassurance to feel stable, they are constantly trying to push back against negative perceptions of themselves and prove that they deserve success; however, this interferes with their ability to communicate with other people. People who are anxious and apprehensive may end up bringing their problems into the workplace and vice versa. Also, the constant pressure and anxiety they experience often damage their mental and physical health.

People with an insecure-ambivalent or "preoccupied" attachment style approach their sexual relationships to **gain reassurance** and approval from their partner. They may also maintain a strategic distance from them to avoid rejection; therefore, although they often appreciate being held and touched, they tend to view sex as a way to get the desired responses of reassurance, happiness, and satisfaction from their partner.

Insecure-avoidant Attachment

The child with an **insecure-avoidant attachment** style has very restrained and seemingly cold emotional displays; the infant does not cry at the time of separation from the mother and tends to avoid her at the time of reunion. These are children who learn very early not to express their needs and not to make requests to the other, **avoid receiving responses of rejection or disinterest from the caregiver (the reference figure), and not** feel the painful frustration that would result from such negative responses. These are children—and they will be adults who do not know how to properly express their anger or needs, showing themselves to be uninvolved and falsely self-sufficient.

Caregivers of children who develop this style of attachment are unavailable, with little or no affection or physical contact with the child, and tend to ignore or reject the child's requests for contact, reassurance, and closeness. In these situations, the child develops an internal operating model characterized by:

- Perception of oneself as unlovable, not deserving of love and attention, incapable of eliciting positive responses of affection and care;

- Perception of the other as unavailable or invasive.

In this case, the behavior is characterized by a marked autonomy and independence and a tendency to maintain a distance from the other, and cyclical behaviors of distancing and rapprochement in the relationship. The **adult** individual with this style of attachment:

- Prefers **cognitive** to emotionality: the person is cold, not very affectionate, detached, and not very inclined to emotional involvement;

- Does not like to get intimately involved in romantic relationships, and always maintains a kind of emotional distance from the other, distracting himself or herself from the couple with outside activities or flirtation;

- Is a cold person who does not attach to the other, avoiding intimacy (not sex) and commitment to the relationship.

  Sometimes boycotts intimacy by choosing partners who are unavailable, unwilling to commit, or engaged in another relationship;

- Has great difficulty perceiving and becoming aware of his internal states, mentalizing them, being accustomed to denying them so as not to see himself rejected.

Because no one taught them as children that their needs can be accommodated and their requests for help or support can be met, adults with this attachment style "don't know how to ask." Thinking that their partners will not be there to help or comfort them:

- Protect themselves by using "deactivation" techniques that allow them to avoid being in the feared position and having to depend on their partner;

- They maintain a strategic distance or lower their feelings and needs for attachment;

- Limit their relationships with other people;

- They avoid conflict and avoid their partners for no apparent reason.

That said, we might mistakenly conclude that people with an insecure-avoidant attachment style are loveless. They are not!

The truth is that they feel love for their partner, which is why they engage in a relationship, but the way they show love and affection can seem cold and indifferent. They are unable to understand their own emotions and are unable to deal with their feelings or past traumas. For example, when their partner does something that irritates them, they try to deny or hide their anger. But unspoken anger doesn't go away! It's just hidden and causes them stress and anxiety.

Disorganized Attachment

According to research, children with a **disorganized attachment style** exhibit inconsistent and contradictory behaviors that are paradoxical, non-purposeful, and disorganized for a purpose; they exhibit **hypervigilance** and a **state of constant alertness** as if there were an imminent danger.

Three types of behavior have been identified that characterize disorganized/disoriented attachment:

- Conflict behaviors;

- Behaviors involving disorientation;

- Behaviors of fear towards the *caregiver.*

Numerous studies have also shown that the child's negative model creates of the main reference figure leads him to avoid requests for help and conflict and not to trust others. The primary state of mind is fear, associated with unresolved losses, fears, and trauma of one or both parents.

Negative self-evaluations and self-loathing characterize the beliefs these children develop; in particular, they will think that they are bad, incompetent, and unlovable; that their parents are unresponsive to their needs, insensitive, and unreliable; and that the world is dangerous and life is not worth living.

This pattern of beliefs leads the child to a sense of alienation from the family and society in general; he will always feel the **need to control others and protect himself** at all times through aggression, violence, anger, and revenge. It is precisely instances of disorganized attachment that lead to the development of aggressive behavior in children and conduct disorders, factors that could then contribute to the development of an antisocial personality.

Adults with a disorganized attachment style choose to stay in the relationship, whether their partner cares for them or not and even when it causes them great pain and psychological damage. They struggle to be emotionally and physically intimate with their partners. Occasionally, this involves using casual sex to satisfy their need for comfort, recognition, and consolation.

After analyzing the different attachment styles, we can therefore conclude that the causes of attachment disorders (insecure attachment) can be varied:

- **Related to the parents:** abuse, neglect, depression or other psychiatric pathologies of the parents, addictions, etc.

- **Related to the child:** temperamental difficulties, premature birth or prenatal or perinatal problems;

- **Related to the environment:** marginalization, poverty, poor living conditions, home or community where violence, abuse, and aggression are experienced.

Attachment style is not a pathology in itself, but it certainly represents an obstacle to a rewarding and effective relationship with important people and, in adults, with the romantic partner.

As we said before going into the analysis of the different attachment styles, there is no such thing as a good and a bad attachment style, but there is the "best" one for you. What is the attachment style that makes you feel safe, secure, and happy with your partner? Regardless of what you have discovered you have, does your partner understand you, and is he or she willing to accommodate you? If the answer is yes, you have found the "best for you" attachment style.

Let's look at how each person's attachment style affects our romantic relationship.

How Does Attachment Style Affect Your Relationship with Your Partner?

Our attachment style affects any aspect of our lives, such as how we choose our partner, how our relationship grows, and even how it ends.

Recognizing our attachment style and that of our partner is critical to understanding our relationship's strengths and weaknesses and understanding what our needs and those of our partner are.

For example, if you both have a secure attachment style, your relationship will be very stable as you are both confident in yourself and each other and can connect perfectly with your partner. In case you have an insecure-ambivalent or avoidant attachment style, you may prefer a partner with a different attachment style than you, but one that meets your needs and makes you feel secure and happy in your relationship. If, however, you are a person with an insecure attachment style and you choose to be in a relationship with a partner with an attachment style similar to yours, you may find yourself in very destabilizing situations if there is not good communication in your relationship because you both need reassurance and this can generate fear and anxiety.

By identifying our attachment style we can identify and understand our needs, our wants, and what we look for in a partner to have a stable and happy relationship; trying to identify our partner's attachment style, instead, we can understand **his** needs, **his** wants and we can strive to show empathy towards him to understand what he feels in certain situations and why he reacts in that particular way. By doing this "exercise" together with your partner and talking openly about what your needs are, you will be able to build an open relationship based on communication.

We are all afraid of being hurt—consciously or unconsciously— and this fear tends to increase when we get what we want. The better a relationship is, the more we fear the "impact of a breakup," and this can generate further anxiety and tension within our relationship.

It's not just poorly handled situations that generate anxiety; the **perceptions** we have of that situation do as well. The same situation may create a mild state of anxiety in one person, but create a panic attack in another.

Some people may become overly possessive of others and experience feelings of jealousy and insecurity when they do not receive the love and attention they desire from their loved ones. Anxiety can cause panic attacks, feelings of fear or overwhelm, and a general sense of unease and tension. It can take over your thoughts and affect many aspects of your existence. If you feel the tension in your relationship, anxiety may be the cause.

Anxiety can put your relationship at risk, regardless of whether you or your partner is experiencing it. In these cases, the advice we give is to undertake a couple or individual path with a psychotherapist. It will allow you to get to know the anxiety, recognize its various symptoms, and understand what it is trying to communicate. This will allow you to have a healthier balance in your relationship. Let's look at how and why anxiety destroys relationships and what you can do to stop it.

How and Why Anxiety Destroys Your Relationship

Some people begin to feel in a state of anxiety, which they perceive as a strong state of discomfort when they enter into an intimate relationship with a stable partner.

Many causes generate anxiety both at the beginning and during a relationship. Some of these are:

- Fear of not pleasing the other person;

- Lack of self-confidence;

- Fear of the "breaking impact" of a good relationship;

- Selfish behaviors of the partner;

- Concerns;

- The person is living in a perverse relationship in which he or she is the victim of manipulation and psychological violence or has experienced past relationships in a state of constant insecurity;

Self-confidence, or lack thereof, is one of the main reasons that generate anxiety in a relationship. For many people, anxiety stems from low self-esteem and the belief that you are not "good enough." Are you afraid that your partner doesn't think you are "good enough"? Do you think your partner may "deserve better"? These feelings of insecurity and inferiority can cause stress and depression. Try talking to your partner about how you feel.

What are some ways that anxiety affects your relationship?

- **BREAK TRUST.** Anxiety causes fear or worry, and this can make you less aware of your true needs at any given time. It can also make you less attuned to your partner's needs! If you're worried about what might happen, it's hard to pay attention to what's happening. When you feel overwhelmed, your partner may feel like you're not there. Anxiety can break trust and connection with your partner.

- **SQUASH YOUR TRUE VOICE.** Anxious people generally have trouble expressing their true feelings. Anxiety can make you believe that something needs to be discussed immediately, when a short pause may be more helpful. If you don't express what you're feeling or what you need, anxiety becomes stronger. Also, if you repress emotions within yourself, they may suck you into an uncontrollable spiral.

- **CAUSES YOU TO BEHAVE SELFISHLY.** People who experience anxiety tend to focus too much on their problems or worries. Your worries and fears could put pressure, stress on your relationship. They may keep you from being compassionate and vulnerable with your partner. If your partner experiences anxiety, you may develop resentment and react selfishly. The attitudes and perspectives we have are contagious. Keeping stress levels under control is especially difficult when your partner is feeling anxious, upset, or defensive.

- **ANXIETY IS THE OPPOSITE OF ACCEPTANCE.** A healthy form of worry will tell you "something is not right" and it comes through that rapid beating of your heart or with that tight feeling in your stomach.

This signal helps you take action, such as when you find yourself defending someone.

Excessive anxiety levels might make you feel like there is a "rock" concert going on in your stomach most of the time. Anxiety makes you reject things that aren't dangerous and avoid things that might benefit you. It also can keep you from taking healthy action to change the things in your life that are hurting you.

- **REPRESENTING JOY.** Experiencing joy requires a sense of security or freedom. Anxiety makes us feel fearful or limited. Also, a brain and body overstressed by anxiety can fail to enjoy sex and intimacy. Negative thoughts and fears affect a person's ability to be present within a relationship, sucking the joy out of it.

Before figuring out what to do with your partner to counteract anxiety within your relationship, you need to understand which of you suffer from it or if you both suffer from it. The next step is to identify the causes of your anxiety. Therefore, it is important to understand anxiety, its triggers, and consequences. Understanding how it manifests itself in relationships can help us detect the negative thoughts and actions that sabotage our love lives. But how can we tell if our partner is insecure?

How to Tell If You or Your Partner Is Insecure

Unlike other disorders that can be diagnosed through lab tests, anxiety is a psychological disorder that can only be diagnosed by identifying its symptoms.

Anxiety is your body's response to triggers such as fear, stress, depression, and traumatic experiences. Early treatment can help sufferers manage this disorder.

People with an insecure attachment type have numerous symptoms of anxiety. Here are some points that can help you identify symptoms of anxiety disorder in you or your partner:

- **NERVOUSNESS.** When you begin a new relationship, you may notice signs of nervousness in you or your new partner. Some tension and nervousness are normal at the beginning of a relationship, certain thoughts or behaviors indicate the presence of an anxiety disorder. Getting angry unnecessarily is a sign of insecure attachment in a relationship. When you decide to argue about an issue that could be amicably resolved, it means that you are not ready to tolerate your partner or that you are fed up with their excesses. Ignoring this behavior can negatively affect the relationship.

- **FEAR OF NOT BEING ENOUGH.** After the courtship phase, you may experience negative thoughts that this new relationship will never be successful or last long because "you're not good enough" or "you don't deserve a happy relationship." The lack of communication coupled with the fear of rejection may make you feel like the entire relationship's weight is on your shoulders and that its success or demise is solely up to you. If you or your partner feels this way, anxiety and stress are creeping into your relationship.

- **LACK OF SELF-CONFIDENCE.** Having low self-esteem and low confidence in yourself and your abilities can allow anxiety to drive a wedge between you and your partner. Self-confidence has a significant influence on a person's ability to build a strong relationship with others, especially romantic partners. If you are a person with low self-esteem, you may feel that you are not good enough for your partner, you may need to be constantly reassured that he/she loves you, and you may begin to be jealous of the people around him/her because you think they are "better than you". If, on the other hand, your partner has low self-esteem, you may find that he/she begins to exhibit jealousy "for no apparent reason"; in reality, he/she just needs reassurance.

Lack of self-confidence breeds **JEALOUSY**. A jealous person is always suspicious of their partner's conduct and all those around them in business and life in general because they fear that they may be left for another person.

Those who are jealous want to spend all their time with their partner and do not want their partner to do things without them. If you are an extremely jealous person or find that your partner is, be very careful. Jealousy puts a strain on your relationship. Being so jealous to the point of demanding all of your partner's time and consideration at the expense of other friendships and relationships can be detrimental to your relationship.

When you question your partner's motives by thinking *"I wonder what he's doing"* or *"I wonder who he's talking to at work"*, *"He's talking to someone very attractive"*, *"He's giving people too much credit"* you are showing that you don't trust him. Your low self-esteem causes a lack of trust in him and the resulting jealousy.

To prevent your relationship from being damaged by the anxiety by low self-esteem in either or both of you, you must strive to be patient with an insecure partner. Try to support him as much as possible and increase his self-esteem. If you feel it is necessary, advise him to seek professional help to resolve his insecurity issues or, perhaps, start this journey together. Your relationship will be much stronger as a result!

- **POOR COMMUNICATION.** The ability to communicate is inherent in human beings. Because of this ability, we can relate to those around us by communicating our thoughts and feelings with them and getting them to do the same with us. However, not all of us have the same communication skills. Some of us are more outgoing, while others are more introverted.

  If in a relationship both partners have difficulty communicating, the relationship will slowly disintegrate. If you don't share your thoughts, feelings, personal problems, past traumas, hopes, or dreams with your partner, you will create a gap between you that, over time, can become a dealbreaker in your relationship. Most misunderstandings in relationships arise precisely because of a lack of communication. Make an effort to communicate with your partner as much as possible!

By doing so, you will be able to solve all kinds of problems and prevent new misunderstandings from arising.

- **LACK OF RESPECT.** Respect must be the basis of any healthy and happy relationship. Disrespecting your partner means being rude to them and ignoring or hurting their feelings. You can disrespect your partner in many ways, both verbally and physically. If you find that, through words and actions, your partner is showing no respect for your feelings, thoughts, or beliefs, try talking to them about it. Pick an appropriate time, keep your cool, and point out to him what behavior you found disrespectful and ask him not to do it again. Don't ignore what happened and the feelings you had at the time. If you don't communicate right away, the disrespect could get worse over time. In the worst-case scenario, those "little" disrespect in the early stages of the relationship can become physical and psychological abuse.

  If, on the other hand, you are the one who has disrespected your partner, don't get upset if your partner points it out. Keep your cool and listen carefully to your partner when they try to communicate with you.

  Take the time to understand why he or she felt hurt, apologize, think about what you can do to improve, and then act accordingly. Remember to always be respectful to your fellow man. This way you can have a happy relationship based on mutual respect.

- **LACK OF CONSENT.** Entering a new romantic relationship sometimes also means the beginning of a new sexual relationship. However, being in a relationship with someone doesn't mean having sex every time you want it or your partner wants it. In a healthy, happy, and successful sexual relationship, it is essential to get consent, respect your partner's boundaries, and enforce your own. Don't force yourself to do something you're not ready for or uncomfortable with. If you respect each other, your bond will be strengthened.

By now you should have figured out not only how to recognize anxiety in all its forms, but also whether you or your partner suffers from it. Before we go over practical ways by which you can relieve stress and the resulting anxiety in a relationship, it is important to first work on yourself. This is the first step in dealing with anxiety within our relationship. We cannot love another person if we do not first love ourselves. If we do not take care of ourselves mentally and physically and meet our own needs first, we are unlikely to understand and meet our partner's needs. It is crucial that you discover the roots of your insecurities and what triggers them in different situations. So let's see how, by working on yourself, you can reduce the toxicity within your relationship.

Chapter 3: Change Yourself to Reduce Toxicity in Your Relationship

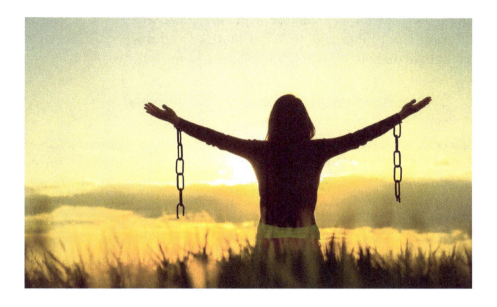

It seems like every day we learn something new about anxiety and the disorders that come with it, and you've probably acquired some information yourself through magazines, books, TV, the Internet, conversations with family members, and/or your doctor. Unfortunately, however, these media outlets view anxiety as something that absolutely must be defeated and describe it as something abnormal. All of this misinformation increases your perception of inadequacy, sense of helplessness, and fragility. Let's debunk some major **myths** about anxiety:

1. Anxiety Problems Are Biological and Hereditary

In part, indeed, anxiety often runs in many families, but this is primarily due to the acquisition of behavioral patterns, not the genes themselves. We may be predisposed to anxiety, but that is different from inheriting it. What matters and makes a difference is what we do every day to control and change our lives.

2. Experiencing Intense Anxiety is Abnormal

Perceiving anxiety is not abnormal; we can all experience it. As we saw in the first chapter, anxiety and fear have their adaptive function; what changes is how we respond to them. For example, through avoidance of situations that may feed or arouse anxiety, we move away from the possibility of experiencing it. It is important to accept these emotions for what they are and use them to take action and continue to do what is important to you.

3. Anxiety is a Sign of Weakness

Anxiety does not make you a weak, unmotivated, lazy person who lacks personality. This idea mainly stems from the fact that we tend to compare ourselves to others and consider what is seen from the outside as representative of the person. We've all met people who seem to have it all together, but have you ever wondered if these people in their intimacy are the same? It is likely that they also have moments of reflection, anxiety, and fear.

What makes the difference is turning those moments into concrete actions and focusing energy, time, and resources in those areas that we can control and change. It's important to understand that you are solely responsible for your actions, and feeling anxiety can be a boost that can help you take concrete action and change something in your life.

4. **Anxiety Can and Must Be Controlled to Live Life to the Fullest**

The moment you try to control your thoughts and emotions to decrease anxiety and feel some sort of relief, you risk having the opposite effect. Controlling your emotions may help you in the short term, but after a while, the anxiety will return and maybe stronger than before. It's important to understand how we can't change our thoughts and replace them with something positive; instead, we need to accept the thoughts and not try to eliminate them.

Managing and Controlling Anxiety

Anxiety is an emotional state that projects us into the future about something that has yet to happen. Unlike fear, anxiety is persistent, so much so that it can occur for days, months, and years because it is fueled by your mind and often not by a real threat or danger. Despite this, it is important to understand that anxiety is an emotional state that helps us, motivates us to achieve the goals we set for ourselves, and steers us away from possible harm.

This chapter will help you change the way you look at things, open yourself up to new possibilities, and bring something new into your life. Remember that "if you keep doing what you've always done, you'll get what you've always gotten." Changing yourself does not mean twisting your personality to fit someone else's. Your personality is part of you. What you can do is learn to manage your anxiety; by doing this, you will be able to manage it within your relationship as a couple. One way you can manage your anxiety is through **Acceptance and Commitment Therapy (ACT),** which can be translated as **Acceptance-Choice-Action**. Let's see what these steps consist of.

1. ACCEPTANCE: involves acquiring skills that can help you respond differently to your fears, anxieties, concerns, and thoughts. The goal of acceptance is to look at them with kindness and try to decrease emotional involvement, making room for what you are experiencing.

2. CHOICE: Choose what direction you want to take your life. What are your values? Who or what is important to you? Choosing to go with your choices and take your direction involves encountering anxiety-related thoughts and physical sensations along the way. You will learn to become friends with them and let them come and go as they please without avoiding them or trying to run away from them.

3. ACTION: what you choose to do to pursue your values and achieve your goals. This will involve commitment and dedication, day in and day out.

At every moment of our lives, we must make choices and we are completely responsible for them. We cannot choose whether or not to feel pain, experience anxiety, and/or worry. But even in this case, we can decide what to do with the thoughts and feelings as they arise and choose what kind of relationship to establish with them.

Try to imagine your anxiety as if it were a person with his personality, character, and manner of dress, and name it. The goal is to imagine the anxiety in a person's form as it arises and try to see it more as a friend rather than an enemy.

The temptation to avoid, suppress and run away from your thoughts can be very strong, but it is important to learn to accept them and establish a relationship of kindness and understanding with them. In the table below you will see some possible scenarios in which you have the power to choose what to do with your worries, anxieties, and fears as they arise:

YOU CAN...	OR YOU CAN...
Observe what your mind says without acting on it.	Do what your mind says.
Meet and accept your thoughts and be with them.	Struggle with them and try to eliminate them.
Observe what your body is doing.	Listen to what your mind says about your body.
Do nothing about thoughts, worries, and feelings.	Try to distract yourself in some way.
Be patient with your thoughts.	Put yourself and others down for it.
Move on with your life.	Fighting with your thoughts and getting stuck.

To better understand how much our thinking affects our actions, let's take a practical example: A guy, who we'll call Simon, is running an errand for work and enters an office building. He walks up to the elevator and thinks, *"Here we go again, here's another elevator. I hate elevators. If I get on it I'll get anxious and possibly have a panic attack. What if someone sees me? What if the elevator gets stuck? I could be locked in for weeks...Maybe it's better to take the stairs."* Simon feels very anxious, changes direction, and takes 15 flights of stairs to get to his destination.

Why did Simon get anxious and go up the stairs? The best answer is, "Simon got anxious."

To better understand, let's consider another version of the same story: Simon is running an errand for work and enters an office building.

He approaches the elevator and thinks, *"The office is on the 15th floor. What if the elevator gets stuck? It is unlikely, and if it does, I will use the internal phone to call for help. No need to worry unnecessarily."* The anxiety subsides and Simon takes the elevator.

In the two versions, **the situation is the same**. What has changed?

- First, Simon's **thoughts** have changed.

- Second, Simon's emotional **reaction** has changed: in the first version, he becomes very anxious, in the second version he remains almost completely calm.

In the first version, Simon's emotional reaction was not due to external factors: it was not the elevator that made him afraid, but his catastrophic thoughts! The real cause is Simon's thoughts, what was said, his so-called internal dialogue.

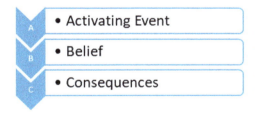

Just as in the alphabet, you don't go directly from A to C without first going through B, Activating events don't cause Consequences without first going through B Thoughts.

Dysfunctional Thoughts

Simon's way of thinking in the first situation is called **dysfunctional**.

A dysfunctional way of thinking does not correspond to reality and does not help achieve one's goals. It is important to realize that dysfunctional thinking is *a habit* and that changing habits takes effort, practice, and practice. Identifying dysfunctional thoughts associated with anxiety is just the first step in changing the way you think. What are the main characteristics of dysfunctional thoughts?

Dysfunctional thoughts can be:

- **Automatic**: they have a lightning-fast onset and are unconscious unless you pay close attention;

- **Distorted**: they do not correspond to the facts, they are inaccurate;

- **Counterproductive**: they cause discomfort and make it more difficult to achieve what you want to achieve;

- **Unintentional**: not chosen and difficult to get away from.

But how can we change the way we think?

Steps to practice at length to more constructively change the way you think are:

1. Identify the thoughts and interpretations of events and situations that cause anxiety;

62 2. Examine thoughts and interpretations to see if they represent a reasonable assessment of reality;

3. Refute dysfunctional thoughts;

4. Find more functional alternative thoughts;

5. Translate the more functional thoughts into behaviors consistent with them;

6. Identify dysfunctional thoughts.

At first, it is not easy to find out what you are thinking about a certain situation because many dysfunctional thoughts become almost automatic. One way to identify dysfunctional thoughts is to start with emotions of anxiety, fear, discomfort, and work backward. To begin with, think about a recent situation in which you felt more anxious or upset than was normal and reasonable. Think back to how you felt and ask yourself the following questions to identify dysfunctional thoughts: *What do I think about myself? What do I think about others? What do I think about the situation? What am I afraid will happen? How do I think about dealing with the situation? What will I do about it?*

Then put your thoughts to the test. One of the best ways to refute dysfunctional thoughts is to write them down on a piece of paper and imagine trying them in court:

would they hold up under cross-examination? Would other witnesses give the same version? It is helpful to ask yourself the following questions to critically examine anxiogenic thoughts:

- *What evidence is there that the thing I fear is really real?*

- *If what I fear happened, would it be important, horrible, unbearable?*

- *Would it have negative consequences for the rest of my life?*

- *How likely is it that what I fear will happen?*

- *What is the worst thing that could realistically happen to me?*

- *What different, alternative ways might there be of looking at things?*

- *Could I interpret the situation differently?*

- *Which of the possible alternatives is more likely?*

- *Which one is more in line with reality and more useful to achieve my goals?*

- *Am I using the wrong ways of reasoning and evaluating reality?*

There are wrong ways of reasoning and evaluating reality that are called **cognitive distortions**. Some of these are:

- **Thinking in terms of all or nothing**. For example, you felt uncomfortable for a moment at a party and decided that the whole experience was a disaster.

- **Generalizing**. Pay attention to words like *always, never, all, none, nothing.* Ask yourself if the situation is that extreme, such as if it's true that *no one* is as shy as you are or that *everyone* thinks you're a failure, or *that everyone will always not accept you.*

- **Mentally filter reality.** You filter reality when you **only** think about your weaknesses, forgetting your strengths. Try to think about the times when you have reported successes, even small ones, and all the resources you have and the things you can do. You also filter reality when you focus only on detail and based on it you come to excessive conclusions, for example, when you don't get the phone call from a friend you were waiting for, you think: *"He doesn't care about me"* or when, if you are for a moment without knowing what to say while talking to someone, you conclude that: *"I never have anything to say."*

- **Belittle**. Devaluing or disqualifying positive aspects. It happens when you underestimate your successes, such as when you tell yourself, *"A child could have done that."*

- **Personalize**. It happens when for no reason, you place all the blame on yourself for something that went wrong or you feel like everyone is looking at you when it's not true, or even when you think, *"I've always jinxed him,"* or *"I ruined his party,"* or *"He's unhappy because of me."* Remember that just as you are responsible for your thoughts and feelings, so are others responsible for theirs. You can influence, but not determine, others' reactions.

- Overestimating the likelihood of an unpleasant event— Risks are often less than you think. How likely is it that what you fear will happen?

- **Catastrophizing**. We often think an event is a catastrophe or that it will have greater consequences for us than it actually will. Ask yourself, *"What difference will it make in a week? What about a year from now? What about ten years from now? Will it still matter to me?"* We often exaggerate the importance of our mistakes and failures.

- **Judging based on emotions**. It happens when you assume that the emotions you feel accurately reflect the facts: *"I feel bad, so things are going wrong"; "I feel anxious, so there must be a real threat."*

- **Jumping to conclusions**. From a detail, you arrive at conclusions, often negative ones, without making the effort to examine the problem in its complexity

- **Mind reading**. This happens when you assume you know what someone else is thinking without asking them or others, e.g., *"I'm sure he thinks I'm a bore and doesn't want to see me anymore."*

- **Being an oracle**. Predicting an uncertain future with certainty. For example, thinking about a speech you have to give in public, you tell yourself, *"I'm sure I'll act like a fool and everyone will laugh at me!"* Just because things have gone a certain way in the past doesn't mean they will be the same in the future.

- **Being too pessimistic**. About the possibility of being able to change a situation. This way of assessing reality is both a cause and a consequence of depression, low self-esteem, weak sense of self-efficacy. There may be no solution, but you will never know unless you try.

One must also be on guard against dysfunctional beliefs that include the verb *must* or similar expressions such as *"It is necessary," "It absolutely must."* It is preferable to use expressions such as *"I Wish", "It would be better", "It is preferable"*.

If you think someone has to do something, i.e., if you demand that they do it, you will most likely be less effective in getting them to do it. If they don't, you will easily incur anger and resentment, unpleasant feelings that will not help you to be as you would like and achieve your goals. For example, instead of telling yourself, *"He should have understood how I felt,"* try telling yourself, *"I wish he would have understood how I felt."*

Refute Dysfunctional Thoughts

Learning to control the thoughts that give rise to and accompany anxiety and think more functionally is key to managing anxiety. Thinking functionally will also help you interpret situations better and reduce the frequency, intensity, and duration of unpleasant emotional reactions. Each of us experiences different thoughts, emotions, and behaviors in different situations throughout the day that affect each other. However, we are often unaware of these mutual influences and the influences of thoughts on emotions. Mostly we think that it is events that directly give rise to emotional reactions.

To refute your dysfunctional thoughts, it is helpful to do the following exercise:

1. Focus your attention on a social situation in which you have felt nervous and uncomfortable, even if not very much.

2. Reflect on how you felt in that situation, the emotions you felt. Try to identify the thoughts you had in that situation, trying to be as complete as possible, that is, to remember everything that went through your mind. You will find that every unpleasant emotion is matched by at least one dysfunctional thought.

3. At this point, start questioning the dysfunctional thoughts and replacing them with more realistic thoughts that are more helpful in achieving your goals.

What you then need to do is change your dysfunctional thinking into **functional** thinking. Functional thinking does not involve rejecting all the negative aspects of life and your behaviors. It consists of **evaluating** things that are both closer to the situation and more helpful in achieving your goals. It is important to distinguish functional thinking from positive thinking, which is overly optimistic and illusory. Let's take an example:

DYSFUNCTIONAL: *"I am sure I will do something wrong. If I don't succeed it will be a disaster!"*

HILARIOUS: *"This time it will be easy, I can't fail. If I fail, I don't care!"*

68

FUNCTIONAL: *"I'm going to try, I'm going to do my best and see how it goes! If it doesn't go well I will be sorry, but I will try to learn from this failure and try again."*

As you deal with dysfunctional thoughts you may have difficulty thinking:

"I feel like I'm thinking about nothing." If you find it difficult to identify the thoughts at first, ask yourself, *"What could be bothering me in a situation like this?"*, *"How could this turn out?"*. With practice, you will be able to identify and challenge your thoughts.

"I can't think of any alternative thoughts." It can be difficult to find different thoughts (from the usual dysfunctional thoughts) that can lead us to change our emotions for the better. However, in the beginning, it may be enough for you to question your old dysfunctional thoughts. It takes time to get good at any skill.

"I have little belief in functional thoughts." You don't need to be convinced, just consider functional thoughts as assumptions to be evaluated and act as if these assumptions are true, and then see what happens.

"I still feel anxious." Until you are completely convinced that nothing terrible is going to happen, you won't be free of anxiety. Still think that you can do it even if you feel anxious. Remember that experiencing some anxiety is normal and have confidence.

Reiterate that having dysfunctional thoughts does not mean wanting or preferring but **demanding**, and thinking that the consequences of not satisfying our desires would be terrible, catastrophic, unbearable, as well as pretending not to struggle and attributing all blame or all credit to others.

Remember that you don't have to fight anxiety, but you do have **to understand it.** Anxiety does not depend on what happens, but on what you think will happen. One way to work on this thinking is to practice emotional journaling. Did you ever keep a journal of your own as a child? If you did, you already know what it is; if you never did, don't worry, we'll explain it to you.

Emotional journaling is an exercise that can make you control your anxiety quickly and easily. Here's how it works: every time you feel anxiety you have to write a page in your diary. First write down the situation, that is, what you are doing while you are feeling anxiety.

Even if what you were doing when you started feeling anxious has nothing to do with the problem you are experiencing badly, write it down anyway. Over time you may notice that certain places, people, times of day are closely associated with anxiety. After you have written down the situation, you need to observe what you are thinking.

Do you negatively imagine something?

Do you expect to experience situations that cause you distress?

Do you think you can't do something well?

Do you fear someone's judgment?

Try to understand what you started to think while you were feeling anxiety and the moment you started to feel it. Observing yourself to understand what you are thinking, how you are anticipating certain threats means getting to know yourself better and starting to take control of your anxiety. This exercise not only makes you focus on your thoughts, analyzing them, and thus loosening the grip of anxiety, but it is the basis for transforming this negative emotion into calm, security, or serenity.

This exercise will allow you to understand that **anxiety is, first of all, a way of thinking**. Only later does it become an emotion. As we have already said, anxiety anticipates a problem that may not be there, so it does not depend on reality; it depends on what you think, or rather, **how** you think.

Like any other emotion, anxiety is the consequence of our thoughts and does not depend on the things that happen to us. Take the time to re-read this chapter several times and periodically do a self-analysis. Has your thinking changed since the last time you read these pages? How many dysfunctional thoughts have you been able to refute? How has emotional journaling helped you realize that anxiety depends on the way you think?

You feel anxiety (and any other negative emotion) if you experience situations that you consider negative.

If starting today, you never judged anything as negative again, and if that were really what you thought (not pretending!), you would no longer feel negative emotions. To get there, you have to start making a very important change, which involves both your language and your view of reality.

From now on, you must eliminate the word "negative"; nothing that happens to you or that you see on television must be negative anymore, but it must become **challenging**.

When you think "negative", it is as if in front of you you see a wall that bars your way, so you cannot go on and you are stuck or blocked. And this is a condition that exposes you to all the negative emotions. On the other hand, when you see things as "challenging", you have a ladder in front of you. This means that no matter how challenging it is, you can continue, you are not stuck, and you can proceed, move forward. If you can transform your idea of what you experience, from the "insurmountable wall" you face when you judge something as negative, to "a strenuous ladder" of challenging situations, the more, the merrier! To accomplish this, you must do two things:

1. Eliminate from your lips (don't say it again!) and from your mind (don't think it again!) the concept of negatively associated with things that happen. Always replace it with "challenging".

2. Do the same thing if others say it. Always think, *"No, it's not negative, it's just challenging!"*

Translate your "challenging" into specific actions. Challenging means it involves commitment and effort: to do what? Identify what commitments the situation you are experiencing entails and turn them into goals. Remember that emotion has nothing to do with what happens, only what you think matters.

If you start to live everything as a challenge in front of any situation, perhaps very demanding, the reality does not change, but you are better, you focus on what depends on you and you act.

Use this method as often as you can. If they don't work the first time, insist a little: when we do something new, we don't always get it right the first time. Insist, give yourself at least a week, 10 days trying every time the anxiety arises. To get rid of it, you have to understand that you need **to change the way you see and live** your life. It is a gradual and continuous inner process. The purpose of these exercises is to make you experience situations differently. It is not enough to block or calm the anxiety, it will come back. You must learn to live and think in a new way if you want to get to the point of eliminating it from your life.

Self-Awareness

An ancient Japanese legend tells of a warlike samurai who challenged a Zen master one day by asking him to explain the concepts of heaven and hell. The monk, however, replied with contempt: "You are nothing but a crude villain; I cannot waste my time with people like you!". Feeling his honor attacked, the samurai became furious and drew his sword, shouting, "I could kill you for your impertinence. "There," replied the monk calmly, "this is hell."

Recognizing that the master was telling the truth about the anger that had invaded him, the stricken samurai calmed down, drew his sword, and bowed, thanking the monk for the lesson. "Behold," the Zen master then said, "this is heaven."

The samurai's sudden awakening and the opening of his eyes to his state of agitation show us how fundamental the difference between being a slave to emotion and becoming aware that it is overwhelming us. At first glance, it might seem that our feelings are obvious; but if we reflect more carefully, we remember all those times that we neglected them too much or became aware of them too late.

To have **self-awareness** or emotional stability is to be aware of your thoughts, what your mental state is like at any given moment, and how well you manage your emotions.

Being aware means being able to be able to recognize about yourself:

- One's needs and desires;

- Your strengths and weaknesses;

- How we react to situations;

- Our emotions and our reactions to them;

- The habits and thought patterns we use;

- One's social preferences; one's tastes.

In particular, self-awareness consists in the *ability to recognize the emotional signals expressed by our body*, to give a consequent name to the emotions that we feel, and that "inform" us on which are the situations in which we feel good and which are those that cause us discomfort. It *is the ability to sense, perceive, recognize and give a name to reality*, as much as possible, in every area and aspect of life.

It seems that practicing self-awareness requires the activation of the neocortex, and in particular the areas of language, which allow us to name awakened emotions. Self-awareness is a neutral mode of mind that supports introspection even in turbulent emotions. Self-observation allows this balanced awareness of passionate or violent feelings. It is the difference between being overwhelmed by a murderous rage toward someone and thinking introspectively, *"There, that's anger I'm feeling,"* even at the very moment we are experiencing it.

In terms of neural mechanics, this subtle shift in mental activity signals that neocortical circuits are actively monitoring the emotion, thus taking a first step in acquiring some control over it. This awareness is the fundamental emotional competence on which all others are based, e.g., self-control.

Being self-aware, in short, means being "aware of both our state of mind and our thoughts about it." Self-awareness can be a form of attention, non-reactive and non-critical, to one's inner states.

This sensitivity can also be less balanced; here are some typical thoughts that reveal emotional self-awareness: *"I shouldn't be feeling this way," "I'm thinking about good things to cheer myself up,"* and, in the case of more limited self-awareness, *"Don't think about it,"* an escape reaction in response to something that upsets us deeply.

Although there is a logical distinction between being aware of one's feelings and taking action to change them, recognizing a deeply negative mood means wanting to get rid of it. However, the recognition of emotions is one thing, and the efforts we make not to act under their impulse are another.

Self-awareness has a more powerful effect on very intense negative feelings: when we say to ourselves, *"There, that's anger I'm feeling,"* this awareness gives us a greater degree of freedom; it gives us the ability to decide not to act on the impulse of anger and even to try in some way to vent it.

Depending on how they perceive and manage their emotions, people can be classified into different categories:

- **Self-aware**: aware of their moods as they arise. They have a clear view of their own emotions, and this can reinforce other aspects of their personality. They are self-reliant individuals who are sure of their limits, enjoy good psychological health, and tend to see life from a positive perspective. When they are in a bad mood, they do not continue to brood and obsess, on the contrary, they manage to get rid of the negative mood before others do. There being attentive to their inner life helps them control their emotions;

- **Overwhelmed**: they are people who are often overwhelmed by their emotions and unable to escape them as if in their mind they had taken over. Being fickle types and not fully aware of their feelings, these individuals lose themselves in them instead of considering them with a minimum of detachment. As a result, realizing that they have no control over their emotional lives, these people do little to escape negative moods. They often feel overwhelmed and unable to control their emotions;

- **Resigned**: although these people often have clear ideas about their feelings, they too tend to accept them without trying to change them. In this category fall two types of subjects:

  - Those who usually have positive states of mind and therefore have little motivation to change them;

  - Those who, despite being aware of their moods, and are susceptible to negative feelings, nevertheless accept them assuming a "laissez-faire" attitude, without trying to change them despite the suffering they bring (for example, people suffering from depression who have resigned themselves to their despair).

We've seen what self-awareness is, but why is it so important to develop it?

Knowing yourself allows you to make predictions about how you will deal with the various situations that life throws at you daily.

By developing self-awareness, you will be able to experience events in a more prepared way. You will have the ability to choose situations, behaviors, and attitudes that are more functional to achieve the goals you have set for yourself. Being more aware also increases the ability to analyze and review events and, consequently, increases the likelihood of distinguishing between the representation of the world that we make to interpret events and experiences and objective reality. Developing self-awareness is important because **things are not as they seem to our senses** at a very rapid and instinctive perception. This ability also helps us to improve our concreteness and effectiveness. But how can we develop self-awareness?

Developing self-awareness is not an easy task. People are so afraid of change that they stick to their old patterns of behavior and attachment styles, even though they bring nothing but pain and loneliness. Start by opening yourself up to the possibility of change.

Self-awareness comes first from self-observation done without judging oneself; to develop it, it is also necessary to train oneself to observe, listen and hear oneself starting with one's sensory perceptions. One way to do this is to answer some simple questions such as:

- *What do I see with my eyes?*

- *What do I hear with my hearing?*

- *What do I feel in my body?*

- *What smell or scent does my sense of smell perceive?*

- *What does what I am experiencing taste like?*

- *What is happening or could happen?*

- *Who else is or will be involved?*

- *Where am I?*

- *Has this happened before? Under what conditions?*

- *What thoughts am I aware of doing at this moment?*

- *What condition is my mind in right now? Calm, agitated, relaxed, concentrated...*

In summary, the awareness of one's "inner world" in the "here and now" can be perceived by asking these four questions:

- *What am I thinking about?*

- *What perceptions do I have?*

- *What emotions am I feeling?*

- *How am I acting?*

Awareness concerns, however, also the knowledge of one's behaviors and habits deriving from our values and from the repetitiveness of mental schemes that can also become real perceptive traps. I could therefore ask myself: "*What do I usually think/try/do when a certain situation arises? How do I act? After a brief reflection, do I act or more often react instinctively?*

By addressing your inner conflicts, you will confront your fears, such as the fear that you don't deserve love, and dysfunctional and destructive thoughts, such as that your partner doesn't care about you. You will then begin to recognize the signs of self-sabotage and eventually eliminates those tendencies from your life.

The path to full awareness may never end, and there are many strategies, techniques, and modalities to reach the higher stages. The fact that it is a very challenging skill does not mean that it is not worth developing, quite the contrary.

In response, you must recognize your share of responsibility when problems arise.

Self-Compassion

The term compassion comes from the Latin: *"cum insieme patior soffro."* Probably the best-known definition is that of the Dalai Lama, who defined compassion as*: "A sensitivity to the suffering of ourselves and others, combined with a deep commitment to trying to alleviate it."*

Many people confuse self-compassion with mindfulness or gratitude. Showing self-compassion means truly **recognizing what it means to be human and what our basic needs are**. Experts say that by fostering compassion for ourselves, we are more readily able to feel it for other people; this means that our kinder, calmer, empathetic approach can radiate outward.

People often show more empathy and compassion toward others than they do toward themselves. When someone we love is hurting, we go out of our way to try to make them feel better by giving them the love and support they need. It is very important to do the same thing for ourselves. The truth is that we cannot be genuinely compassionate for other people until we first learn to be compassionate for ourselves. But how do we do that?

Showing self-compassion toward yourself doesn't mean buying chocolates and enjoying them in a time of trouble; it doesn't even mean simply being "nice and kind**.**"

It means treating yourself with love and support when you feel pain, disappointment, or inadequacy. Instead of condemning and judging yourself for feeling this way, you need to accept the way you feel and understand that there is nothing wrong with that.

Many people will argue that self-compassion will only cause people to become complacent, self-satisfied, or selfish.

They may believe that being kind to yourself means never taking responsibility for your mistakes.

This couldn't be further from the truth. Showing self-compassion does not mean giving up the consequences of your actions.

We all experience similar emotions, such as pain and disappointment, and we all have our shortcomings and flaws. If you reflect on this, you will understand that all your problems are simply part of being human and that these challenges do not imply that there is anything wrong with them. Being more human will help us form stronger bonds with other people, including our partners. Also, you will be able to handle any conflict with the people around you in a healthy way that leads to a happy and lasting relationship.

Compassion can be hard, it can mean setting boundaries, being honest, and not willing to give ourselves and others what they want, but rather what they need. For example, an alcoholic wants another drink, but it is not what they need.

Self-compassion is a way of coping with painful experiences, feelings that scare us, or memories of past trauma. Instead of avoiding painful emotions or trying to suppress them, self-compassion teaches us how to deal with what causes us pain. But how can you develop self-compassion?

- **Find a balance with your inner voice.** Negative inner dialogue is not evidence of something "wrong" with us that needs to be fixed. It is a characteristic of being human.

Our complex cognitive system, capable of imagining, anticipating ... is just as prone to dwell on negative thoughts like *"If only I had ..." and "I should have ..."*. This triggers the internal/external threat-protection system. "Self-compassion is always a trade-off with self-criticism." For some people, the balance is so unbalanced that their inner critic rules who and how they are in the world. Not only is this a miserable existence, but it often underlies problematic relationships with drugs, alcohol, food, or work in an attempt to find relief, as well as mental health issues, including depression.

- **Find the source of thoughts.** Many of us have become adept at avoiding unpleasant emotions. This is because we are distracted by our hectic lives or are simply unable to cope and manage what we might discover. The first step toward self-compassion is **to become aware** of our inner world:

  - What causes us feelings of anger, disgust, or shame;

  - How we instinctively react to these emotions;

  - The content of our internal dialogue;

  - Any blocks or resistance we encounter.

- **Become a keen observer of yourself.** This process may be difficult, especially for people who have experienced trauma, who may have absorbed their attacker's words into their internal dialogue.

Developing self-compassion is the ability to feel safe instead of traumatized, developing flexibility in your mind so that you have a compassionate mind.

- **Dialogue with your inner voice.** In your mind, there is a part of you that is attacking, angry and hostile, and there is another part of you that is receiving the criticism and feeling upset and hurt. So it's a matter of imagining your inner dialogue like that of two strangers on the street and describing their relationship. As soon as you can see it as outside of you, you can see it more clearly. It can also shed light on your inner critic's origins by recalling your dynamic with a parent, teacher, or colleague.

- **Treat yourself as you would a friend.** When you're going through a hardship, try telling yourself, *"It's not that bad," "It'll be okay," "Look on the bright side."*

Compassion has as much to do with our relationships with other people as it does with ourselves. Fostering connections and ways we can care for others is important. When we feel supported by others and safe, we are more likely to feel compassion toward others and give them support. The goal is to create a "compassionate mindset" where we not only feel compassion for ourselves and others but are also open to receiving it.

Self-compassion and self-awareness are crucial techniques to practice if you want to have a successful relationship.

They can help you understand your conflicts and deal with them consciously and humanely, allowing you to finally have the relationship you deserve. Learning to be compassionate requires daily discipline and commitment. The hardest part is permitting yourself to do so and accepting that you deserve to be at peace with yourself. Making this commitment marks the beginning of a "permanent journey." Who do you want to be accompanied by on this journey? Do you want to take your self-critic or your compassionate friend with you?

Remember that the purpose of anxiety is to get you to take action to reduce it, but this can have the opposite effect and lead you to increase it. You must take action. By deciding to take action, you will control your life and decide what direction to take it.

How Grief Can Change People in a Relationship

Emotional pain can cause anxiety disorders and depression in people. Instead of getting help from someone to deal with their problems, these people decide to turn to drug use, compulsive shopping, extreme sports, or become immersed in their work. None of these, of course, is a good solution to their problems; on the contrary, they add more problems to their existing ones in many cases.

If you've been hurt in the past, maybe you're afraid to open yourself up to new experiences. Maybe you had absent or neglectful parents as a child, you were bullied at school, or your partner cheated on you.

Whatever your past hurts are, they could affect your life in the present; they could make you a more closed-off person who is reluctant to put himself in a position where he will be vulnerable again. We all experience pain, disappointment, stress, and loneliness at different times in our lives. When you accept the possibility of experiencing these feelings, you are admitting that you are human. It's natural not to want to be hurt and feel pain, but avoiding new experiences out of fear means missing out on possibilities; you may miss out on the chance to be truly happy and experience meaningful moments in your life.

Indeed, it's not easy, however, you should allow yourself to let your guard down and be vulnerable with the people you love and who love you. By overcoming your past hurts (with the help of those who love you or an expert), you will have healthy and happy relationships with other people. Like all things, this process takes time. Be patient with yourself, gain self-confidence, and practice self-awareness and self-compassion. By heeding the advice in this chapter, we are confident that you will succeed. By working on yourself, you will be able to take back control of your life. Let's see how.

Taking Control of Your Life

No one chooses of their own accord to experience anxiety on themselves, but every moment you spend controlling anxiety is a moment that takes you away from living life as it matters to you.

Imagine you are pulling a rope against a monster (the monster represents your anxiety);

you have one end of the rope and the monster has the other and there is an endless chasm between you. You hold and pull the rope from your side, trying to beat the monster who wants to take you into the abyss, but he pulls harder and harder too. So you get stuck in the fight against anxiety, you can't turn your attention to anything else or use your hands to do what you like. There is only one way to overcome this challenge: you have to let go of the rope that keeps you tied to the monster, to your suffering. By letting go of the rope you can begin to take back your life and your freedom without waiting until you have defeated the monster. How can you do this?

Acceptance and Commitment Therapy (ACT)*, Acceptance-Choice-Action,** and ***Mindful Acceptance will help you have an alternative and encourage a shift in perspective from common understandings of anxiety and fear.

Mindful Acceptance is an active, fully conscious, and gentle attitude toward your mind, body, and life experience. Mindful Acceptance includes **compassion,** which is defined as a sensitivity to one's own or others' suffering, accompanied by a desire to alleviate it. In this case, it is like compassion in action, as it allows you to cultivate your ability to accept the severity of your judgmental mind and emotional suffering with gentleness and compassion. Acceptance means *noticing and knowing* what you experience, and it doesn't mean you have to like the latter. Jon Kabat-Zinn, the inventor of the *Stress Reduction Clinic* at the University of Massachusetts Medical School, encapsulated in one sentence the true essence and main qualities of mindfulness: *"paying attention, intentionally, in the present and without judgment."*

Paying attention means being able to get more in touch with yourself and your life circumstances, learning to listen to yourself to grow and contact your vitality. To pay attention, you must **choose** to do it, decide to do it intentionally, cultivate and learn to do it day after day, trying to stay focused in the present. The present is what matters; staying focused on the here and now is very difficult, as the mind can very easily start to wander and go somewhere else.

It is important to learn to live and be in the present because it is the only space we can experience. All of this has to be done in a **non-judgmental way**, one of the most difficult qualities to learn, as we always tend to judge and evaluate what we do. We're not saying don't judge, as our mind will always lead us to judgment, but what you can do is **accept** and notice judgment and see it as just a thought and not something that defines who we are and what we want from our lives.

But how to be able to do this? We suggest you try mindfulness exercises. The purpose of mindfulness exercises is to focus on the breath because thoughts and feelings and the breath are constantly changing. Breathing exercises help you pay attention to and focus on your breath while simultaneously letting the thoughts and feelings come and go without getting stuck there with them. You choose what and how to pay attention to, and you are the one who decides what to do. Let's see how.

1. Feeling Your Body and Mind: Acceptance

One of the basic steps to being able to "let go of the rope" is to learn to feel your body and thoughts for what they are and not as judgments that represent who you are.

Before you can do this, you are bound to encounter difficulties but don't give up. When we do something new, not everything succeeds at first go! Sometimes you need to try again and again, but you will reach your goals with perseverance and determination. To get what you want in life you have to open yourself up to the possible difficulties that may arise and this can only be done by stopping avoiding pain at all costs.

Mindful Acceptance exercises are meant to help you live your life to the fullest and can help you increase your ability to observe the changes in your body as anxiety arises and try to meet your unpleasant sensations with kindness and compassion without trying to avoid them and fight what your body is doing. The goal is to be able to convert what you see as a difficulty and discomfort-into something vital.

2. Don't Listen to Everything Your Mind Says

The mind is constantly at work and is constantly producing thoughts. It is these thoughts, the moment you listen to them, that tends to trap you! Don't listen to everything your mind says, but learn to watch your thoughts without conflicting with them. Depending on how you use your thoughts, your mind can either be your ally or your worst enemy. Ask yourself, *"If I listen to what my inner voice is suggesting, will I bring change to my life?"*, *"Will it bring me closer to my values? What has my past taught me?".*

These are important questions and if the answer is no, but you obey what your mind is saying, this will lead to you being stuck in your anxieties, worries, and fears.

3. Choose the Values That Guide Your Life

Values are everything important to you and only to you. What do you do to live your life in alignment with your values?

It is not easy to find and express your values, but you can start by thinking about areas of your life that you consider important, such as family, relationships, friends, work, and self-care. Focus on each of these areas to identify your values and what is truly meaningful to you. Think about what is important to you and ask yourself: do my values represent something really meaningful to me or are they the result of what I have learned is right to do? Values are not rules to follow, but a light that guides us toward the life we want to have. Your worries, anxieties, and fears may be an obstacle to your values, but they could also be signs that you are moving in the direction of what is most valuable to you. Ask yourself what your values are and if your thoughts are somehow blocking your action.

4. Achieve Your Goals: Take Action

Unlike values that last a lifetime, goals are short-lived; once achieved, a goal no longer exists. To live a life in line with your values, you need to set small goals that, day after day, accompany you along the direction you have chosen to take your life. But how do you set goals and achieve them? Below are 5 steps:

- Specificity: you need the goal to be something concrete;

- Significance: the goal must reflect something that is important to you and reflects your values;

- Activity: choose a goal that you are capable of achieving and that can add energy and vitality to your life;

- Realistic: choose a goal that is achievable about your life circumstances;

- Timing: set a goal so that you can accomplish it on the day, time, and place you have scheduled it.

These steps show the importance of your goal being something achievable and doable about the context that characterizes your life. Don't set big unattainable goals. Set small, short-term goals and achieve them. Achieving them requires continuous commitment and dedication. Achieving your goals is not always easy, there will be times when you feel lost and think that everything you do is useless. Don't beat yourself up! If you get lost during your journey, you can go back and start over.

These four tips will help you have an alternative and incentivize a shift in perspective from common knowledge about anxiety and fear. Through the *ACT and Mindfulness* approach, we have tried to show you how common ideas about anxiety and fear, and the thoughts and feelings that come with them, act as barriers that do not allow you to take action and enact changes in your life.

Your values will allow you to make the changes necessary to achieve your goals and accomplish what is truly important to you and important to you.

Remember that it is not an easy path, it will take time and you will often find yourself lost along the way, but with commitment and dedication, in small steps, you will be able to achieve your goals and live a full life in line with your values.

In this chapter, we debunked some false myths about anxiety, saw how you can learn about it, understand it and manage it by working on your thoughts, gaining self-awareness and self-compassion, and delved into some strategies you can apply to regain control of your life. We all can handle stressful events more than we sometimes imagine, and some self-control techniques enhance these abilities. To recap, what are the steps to take if you find you are suffering from anxiety?

1. **IDENTIFY THE CAUSE.** As we have seen, the first thing to do if you suffer from anxiety is to identify the specific situation that is causing it.

2. **NOTE THE PROBLEM.** After you have identified the situations that contribute to your anxiety attacks or panic attacks, write down the problem and try to be very specific in your description, including what is happening to you, where, how, with whom, why, and what you would like to change.

3. **FIGURE OUT HOW TO SOLVE THE PROBLEM.** Draw up as many options as possible for solving the problem. Consider the likelihood that these options will help you solve the problem. Select the option you feel is most appropriate. Develop a plan to try the chosen option and try to implement it. If you don't get results with the option you chose and implemented, remember that you have other options to use. Then go back to the list and select the next preferred option.

4. **BREATHING EXERCISES**. When anxiety or panic attacks come, you begin to breathe more rapidly. This rapid breathing creates unpleasant feelings, such as agitation, lightheadedness, and mental confusion. Learning a breathing technique to slow it down can relieve your symptoms and help you think more clearly. The following technique is a practical remedy that can help you stop the agitation and fear of the moment and reduce the symptoms of anxiety:

   - Breathe in through your nose and count 3 seconds by saying, "one, two, three."

   - Always exhale through your nose, and again count to three, saying, "RELAX, two, three."

   - Repeat the exercise for two to three minutes and then breathe normally. Your breathing will have become regular again!

This breathing technique can be used to slow down your breathing whenever you feel anxious anywhere and without anyone else noticing. They seem like trivial activities, but you will find out how different methods on how to relax are important pillars to fight anxiety in unpleasant situations.

5. **RELAXATION TECHNIQUES.** Knowing how to release muscle tension is an important treatment for treating anxiety. Relax and you will have a general feeling of calm, both physical and mental.

6. **MANAGING THOUGHTS.** Thought management exercises are useful when you are troubled by constant or recurring distressing thoughts. Alternatively, you can learn "mindfulness techniques" to redirect your attention from negative thoughts to positive ones. We replace disturbing thoughts by making reassuring self-disclosures. The choice of thought management technique will depend on the type of anxiety.

7. **LIFESTYLE CHANGE.** Change your lifestyle; take part in an enjoyable daily activity. It doesn't have to be anything super demanding or expensive. Just small things you like to do to take your mind off your worries. Have you ever considered relaxing activities like adult coloring books? These activities can reduce tension.

8. **INCREASE EXERCISE.** Regular exercise helps reduce anxiety by providing a way to eliminate the stress that has built up in our bodies.

9. **REDUCE CAFFEINE INTAKE.** Caffeine is a stimulant, and one of its side effects is to keep us alert and perhaps a little too awake! It also produces the same physiological response of arousal that is triggered while we are under stress. Reducing the amount of coffee per day will reduce anxiety.

10. **REDUCE ALCOHOL INTAKE.** Many people resort to alcohol to deal with stress, anxiety, and depression. In reality, once the effect wears off, the anxiety and depression attacks will always be there. Alcohol is not a way to reduce anxiety.

11. **IMPROVE TIME MANAGEMENT.** Make sure you have planned time for rest and some activities to do in your free time! The day is not made up of 48 hours! Turn down the pace and set aside moments of calm and relaxation.

We are confident that by putting into practice the tips in this chapter, you will manage your anxiety and regain control of your life. After doing this inner work, you will be able to stop anxiety from intruding into your relationship. In the next chapter, we will see how.

Chapter 4: Basics for a Successful Relationship

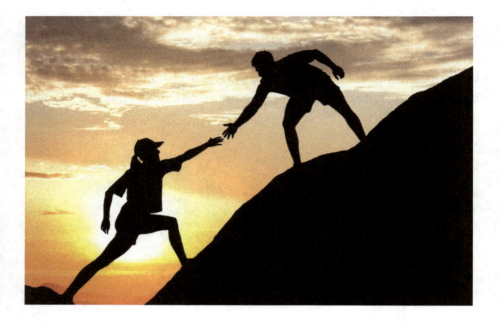

We can compare a relationship to an airplane trip. For the trip to be successful, the pilot and co-pilot must work together. Do you know why both are necessary? The answer is quite simple. The workload on an airplane is very high. The first reason for having two pilots in the cabin is to reduce the workload on one person and thus ensure passenger safety. In the division of tasks in the cabin, the two pilots are divided into Pilot Flying and Pilot Monitoring.

The Pilot Flying has to take care of the aircraft and navigation; he has his hands on the controls, takes off the aircraft, monitors the position of the aircraft concerning the route, and makes sure that it is flying well and following the correct route, altitude and speed. On the other hand, Pilot Monitoring takes care of the communication with the tower and monitors the aircraft's systems such as the engine, hydraulics, electronics, and makes sure everything is working as it should. Another reason why they are both necessary is that if a problem arises, such as an engine failure, only one of the two pilots would notice it; this is because one has his attention focused on the flight and his gaze is almost fixed on the navigation screen, while the other has his gaze on the engine screen in addition to the navigation screen.

How can we apply this example to our relationship? Successful relationships require that both partners strive to do their best, understand the other, be patient, honest, and respectful. If we do this, we can have a successful relationship and our "journey" will be smooth despite the turbulence of life. We must always be careful that anxiety does not "fail the engine" of our relationship. In this case, at least one of you must recognize the symptoms of anxiety so that you can intervene as soon as possible and regain control of your relationship. But how do you find the right romantic partner? The first thing to do is to set your goals. Let's see how.

Establish Your Relationship Goals

Romantic relationships are a challenge for everyone.

No matter how many great couples you see on social, no matter how many loving hugs and kisses photos you see of your friends, no intimate relationship is without its problems. We all have an innate need for love, care, and attention, and when these needs are not met, we experience emotions of anger and sadness. You must keep in mind that your partner cannot meet all of your needs in a relationship, just as you cannot meet **all** of his or her needs. With that in mind, there will inevitably be times when you feel unloved, uncared for, misunderstood, hurt and angry!

What will ensure longevity in your relationship is **how** you and your partner handle the conflicts that arise during your relationship. However, to succeed in this, you need to choose a partner who will work with you to build a long and satisfying relationship. But what do you need to do to find a romantic partner with whom you can successfully cooperate and have a successful relationship?

1. **First of all, clear your mind.** The first step in finding the ideal mate is to take a pen and paper. Of course, you don't have to write a personal ad. What you need to do is ask yourself what you want and need. Entering into a relationship just to not be lonely is not a strong enough foundation for any kind of relationship. Before you meet someone new, you should try to look objectively at what kind of person would be right for you. To succeed in this, you can write a list of your qualities and those you desire in your ideal mate.

   This list should include: your personality traits and those of your ideal mate, and the same for physical characteristics, interests, hobbies, religion, and beliefs, if you want children and if you can accept a man who already has children, your way of communicating, etc.

Maybe you can get help from your friends to help you. Maybe you can get friends to help you outline your side and use what you've learned in your past relationships. If you use this method, it will be easier to recognize your most compatible personalities. We have already talked about attachment styles. You must recognize yours so that you can be as honest as possible when compiling your list.

2. **Turn the list into a profile of the person you are looking for.** It doesn't have to be a list of demands, but it should help you understand what you are looking for in a partner. It must be realistic and based on priorities.

   Studies have shown that women rate: personality, sense of humor, common interests, intelligence, cleanliness, appearance, sensuality, getting to know a man through a friend, voice, spirituality, profession, money, talent, and finally religion; while men rate: personality, sense of humor, intelligence, common interests, appearance, cleanliness, sensuality, voice, talent, spirituality, money, religion, getting to know a woman through a friend, and finally, profession.

3. **Love yourself and your body.** Your ideal mate will be the person who loves you for who you are and wants you to do the same. Work on your self-esteem so that you don't hang on to his every word.

   To succeed at this, make a list of all the good things about yourself, such as what makes you a fabulous friend, what are your 10 accomplishments, what you are proud of in life, etc.

4. **Don't be too picky**. You're not setting up a computer! You and your ideal mate are looking for someone to get to know and make happy. Get to know as many people as you can in various settings, keeping your attachment style and what you're looking for in your partner in mind. Show an open attitude to those little details where you and the other person can improve or compromise. If you're fixated on a specific list of attributes, you'll probably never find that person. Because of this demanding attitude, you risk pushing someone away or even getting a relationship off to a late and bad start.

5. **Remember that your past experiences, your childhood, the way you grew up will influence your relationship**; so, if you haven't yet, identify your attachment style and identify your ideal match based on your role models and core beliefs.

6. **Ask yourself questions as you get to know a new person better**. As the relationship evolves and the two of you grow closer, how can you find out if this person is the one? Love can confuse you and cause you to overlook little things that could turn out to be much bigger once you start a life together.

Things to find out before determining that this person is the one are:

- *Is he moody or hiding things from you that you should know instead?*

- *Are there any financial issues? A difference in financial availability or economic problems can cause a lot of grief, so honesty on this subject is essential.*

- *Do you get along well together for long periods?*

- *How does he behave with his and your family?*

- *Is he respectful, dismissive, interested, bored?*

- *Is his reaction a problem for you?*

- *Are you of the same opinion as far as the talk of children, career?*

All of these things are so important! Don't settle! If you find that he is not the person for you, don't get attached to him or try to convince yourself that he will improve or that you are too demanding. You know what you want in a partner (you wrote it in the previous passages). Be careful not to demand perfection, though!

7. **Observe the family situation of your "hypothetical" partner.** Look at how the parents treat each other and try to understand what they expect from you. While this doesn't do justice to all the personal work a person might have done on themselves, it can help you understand the family context in which your partner lived and their attachment style.

If the person you'd like as your romantic partner has a history of abuse, look at how they deal with children, animals, weaker people, or their subordinates, or how they act in times of stress and conflict. Many people with such a past become strong and kind, while others repeat the sick pattern they suffered.

Get to know his friends, too. The social context may let you know that she is not the right person for you.

8. Never try to change someone into your ideal partner.

By now you should be clear in your mind what your goals are. What you need to do now is to examine what you need to look for in a partner and how you can do it.

What to Look for in a Romantic Partner

We have seen what you can do to find a romantic partner. Looking for a romantic partner means looking for a like-minded person with whom you can not only share your life but who can bring out the best in you. You will have interacted with many people throughout your life and sometimes even started romantic relationships with some of them.

You may have become infatuated with someone you considered very attractive and started a relationship. At first, it always seems like there are no problems, then when difficulties arise, you find out how love affects your daily life and how you and your partner react to situations, stress, and anxiety. Unfortunately, many times these relationships end due to a lack of compatibility.

But is there a way to increase your chances of finding the right person without trying too hard? Yes. When you apply mindfulness to your search for your "ideal" partner, your chances of finding the right person for your increase.

In the previous chapter, we saw what self-awareness and self-compassion are and how to cultivate them; if you make an effort to put into practice what you have learned so far, you will undoubtedly find your ideal partner. But what are the **qualities** to look for in a partner?

Plato said:

> *"Choose someone better than you as a partner. You don't need someone who loves you the way you are. You need someone who will help you grow every day. True love is admiration, so the partner you choose should have those qualities you lack. If the two of you are committed to helping each other grow, you will take the stormy periods of any relationship as opportunities to grow with each other. That's why the right person for you is not just someone who accepts you, but someone who makes you develop your fullest potential in this life."*

For a partner to be there and help you get through difficult and dark times in your relationship without running away in the face of the smallest difficulties, they need to have several qualities. Of course, it cannot be only your partner who has these qualities. You must have them as well. If you find during the reading that you don't have them, make an effort to cultivate them yourself. As we said at the beginning of this chapter, a relationship is like an airplane ride; to arrive at your destination safely, both partners must **work together**. The right romantic partner is the one who helps you boost your self-esteem and supports you by working together on your relationship. Let's look at some important qualities to possess, cultivate and look for in each other:

COMPATIBILITY. The first thing to look for in the "ideal" partner is compatibility. This may seem obvious, but it's not. Have you ever pretended to like something the person you're interested in likes just to impress them? Well, this is not a good strategy. For a relationship between two people to work, you need to have things in common and mutual interests. If the person you like likes to visit museums, and you just to impress them pretend to like them, you will find yourself reluctantly going to the exhibits just because during the acquaintance you pretended to like them.

Don't lie about your interests! You don't have to have **every** interest in common, just a few will do. However, engaging in activities together, finding time to discuss, and setting goals for your relationship while figuring out how to resolve conflicts is crucial for a relationship to work.

EMPATHY. Empathy is the ability and willingness to put yourself in other people's shoes and imagine how they are feeling. Without the ability to empathize, treating you with compassion, kindness and consideration will probably not be a priority.

SENSE OF HUMOR. When relationships are strained, humor can spread a sense of challenge and turn a moment from bad to good.

APPRECIATION. For your relationship to be strong and long-lasting, it's not enough for you or your partner to be romantic and passionate. You must show appreciation for each other for who you are. How to do this. You should both make an effort to get to know each other better, truly understand each other, and accept not only the good qualities but also the flaws.

SUPPORT. We all face difficult times throughout our lives, and it is precisely in these moments that we need to have support and understanding from our partners. If one of you has a problem, instead of supporting each other, one of you pulls away and this gap is not resolved, the relationship may begin to fail. The more we pull away from our partner, the more lonely, neglected, and abandoned we feel; over time, this way of doing things can be one of the causes of the end of our relationship.

GOOD COMMUNICATION SKILLS. Two people who love each other and are motivated to together have the power to resolve all conflicts. Working through conflicts together, however, requires time, patience, and skillful communication.

People who are good at expressing themselves and listening to others are much more likely to understand and support you and maintain healthy relationships. It is important to find **common ground** and **compromise**. There can be many steps to come to terms with each other until you both feel heard, which is exactly why it takes a while to resolve conflicts. Usually, good listeners and communicators are better at identifying and addressing their feelings.

Talking implies **clarifying the problem, understanding its deeper meaning** and importance, making sure that each partner understands the other's position, **taking into account the emotions** each feels; it also implies showing empathy for the other and discussing until a solution is reached that you feel is right for both of you. Problems should be discussed until both people feel better.

UNDERSTAND EMOTIONS. Emotions are part of human nature and are strongest and most intense when we are happy and angry. When we face an argument or discuss our partner's emotions, the emotions that prevail are the negative ones, but what makes the difference is **the way we react**. Some people react immediately by going along with their impulses, and in this way, discussions degenerate. Others, on the other hand, stop and think before acting. This second option is best because thinking before acting allows us to control our reactions. A partner who understands the other person's emotions strives to understand them understands when the other person is angry and tries to help them without attacking or offending them.

ESTABLISHES GROUND RULES. Usually, at the beginning of a relationship, things are always "roses and flowers" but, when the courtship period ends, differences and disagreements begin to emerge. Before this happens, it would be wise to establish some basic communication rules together; this will help you to discuss things constructively.

For example, you may decide to make it a goal to speak in a calm voice when a conflict of opinion is about to arise rather than shouting at each other; not to roll your eyes at each other; avoid walking away in the middle of an argument, threatening divorce, making your partner jealous, belittling them with insults, or being physically aggressive.

The goal of these ground rules is to anticipate conflict and arguments and be prepared to limit the damage (if there should be any).

This way, you will learn from each other what to do when you are feeling bad, sad, angry, and how to meet your partner's needs when they are feeling the same way.

ASK FOR AN EXCUSE. Sometimes this little 5-letter word seems hard to say. Self-awareness will help you and your partner perceive yourself and your actions objectively; through this, you can recognize your flaws, admit mistakes, and understand and forgive your partner's missteps.

BE READY. We left it for last but not because it is less important than the other characteristics.

If you've analyzed the person you like in light of all the characteristics we've listed and you think you've found your ideal partner, there's one last question you need to answer: *is he/she ready for a serious relationship?* Committing to a relationship means taking time away from yourself to dedicate to another person, committing time and energy, and taking responsibility.

Examining these qualities will help you find your romantic partner and also be a good match for him/her.

Another aspect to consider when choosing a partner is attachment styles which we have already discussed in the previous chapters. You don't need to have the same attachment style as your partner; the key thing is that you are both willing to accept the peculiarities of the other. For example, if you have realized that your attachment style is preoccupied while your partner is avoidant, you must first accept each other's peculiarities and you both need to work hard on your relationship;

if you need a lot of reassurance, your partner must understand that and be willing to give it to you, while you will strive to understand that it is difficult for your partner to express his feelings because of his past, but that does not mean that he does not love you and that he would not do anything to meet your needs. Regardless of whether your partner's emotional closeness requirements match your own, consider whether you feel supported by him when you express your needs to him or whether you're sacrificing those parts of yourself for the sake of your relationship.

If, on the other hand, you've noticed that your attachment style is avoidant, you should keep in mind that your natural detachment could confuse or even hurt your partner, especially if the latter has a preoccupied attachment style. You might think that only a person with the same attachment style as you can really understand you and thus get to enter into a relationship with them. Be very careful, however. If you are in a relationship with someone as independent and emotionally closed off as you are, it could end up making you feel even more alone.

When facing difficult times, everyone needs to turn to someone for comfort and support.

If you aren't willing to be a support for your partner, this could drive you apart because he may seek the support he needs from someone else who is willing to listen. Having a reliable partner who can offer comfort, help, and relief from life's inevitable difficulties can be a real blessing.

If you're not very empathetic and don't have good communication skills, strive to improve in this respect. On the other hand, if you feel that your partner is not supportive, instead of turning to someone else when you feel stressed, explain clearly but calmly what your needs are and ask if they can make an effort to listen to you with interest. This will bring you closer together. Having a partner who listens to you when you face difficulties is having a "port in the storm."

In addition to supporting you through difficult times, you and your partner must support each other in dreams. If you had a dream in your drawer that you wanted to achieve before you met, don't give up on it! Pursuing your desires or even just figuring out what they might be is important to feeling fulfilled in life.

If you and your partner support each other by encouraging each other to pursue your dreams, your relationship will be healthy and stable and you will grow closer because your partner will become your right-hand man.

While we've talked about the characteristics to look for in an "ideal" partner, you may have noticed that it's not enough for him or her alone to have them. Many people worry about finding a partner who meets all their needs and has all the qualities mentioned above, but they don't worry about being good partners for each other in turn by cultivating the same qualities.

If you want a partner who will give you all this, you must be willing to do the same thing in return. To have a stable relationship, you both must have these qualities or at least make an effort to cultivate them.

For a relationship to work, it is important to meet each other halfway, make compromises, sometimes be accepting, and be tolerant of the other. In this way, your relationship will be a haven for both of you and a harbor during the storms of life. We've gone over in broad strokes what qualities both you and your romantic partner must-have for your relationship to be stable and lasting. Now we're going to look at some aspects in more detail. Let's start with communication.

Communication to Achieve a Successful Relationship

We live in a world where communication has become really easy. Technology allows us to be in touch with people on the other side of the world and know what is happening in different countries. But does communicating just mean exchanging information?

We are so used to using social networks that sometimes we find it hard to establish "real" relationships and have "real" friends. By now we have become accustomed to sending instant messages and reducing our emotions to simple emoticons: a crying face if you're sorry and a sad face if you're happy (maybe at that moment something doesn't even make you laugh, but you put that face on anyway). So what does it mean to communicate?

Communicating means: *"to transmit something to someone", to make them participate in mental or spiritual content, in a state of mind, in an often privileged and interactive relationship.*

To communicate with someone means to relate, to have a relationship of "dependence", participation and understanding in a mutual way.

Communication is the basis of relationships. It can be learned and improved, starting from a reflection on one's way of acting and relating to others. It is important to become aware of our communication, its effects on us, our interlocutors, and our relationships to transform it into effective communication. Having good relationships with those around you and especially with your chosen partner is critically important to have or learn to cultivate good communication skills. People with poor communication skills are much more likely to have unresolved arguments and unhealthy relationships. On the other hand, if you can establish a good, open channel of communication with your partner, you will be able to build a long-lasting and happy relationship. If you and your partner can't find a balance in the way you communicate, you may always be defensive during an argument.

Instead of focusing on the problem and ways to solve it, the only thing you will think about is coming out victorious from the conflict by being right!

Remember that how you and your partner communicate with those around you depends a lot on your attachment style, how you grew up, past life experiences, etc. However, this should not serve as "justification".

The experiences you have had, although painful, are indeed "past" and continuing to have the same views over time can only cause problems in the relationship between you and your partner.

Don't get stuck on the old methods of communication you've used throughout your life, adopt new ones!

How can you create a good communication bridge between you and your partner?

We have already mentioned that it is useful to establish rules together at the beginning of a relationship. For example, you and your partner can decide together to speak to each other respectfully without raising your voice. This will be of great help to you when problems arise and you have to deal with an argument. If you have established from the beginning to keep calm, have a calm tone of voice, and not attack each other with barbs and sarcastic tones, it will be much easier for you to communicate healthily.

Of course, communicating doesn't mean that you always have to be the one to talk about how you're feeling, your problems, and your emotions.

You must do, but it's of equal importance that you listen carefully to your partner when he or she is the one who needs your support. If your partner talked about their problems every day, how their day went, but wasn't willing to listen to yours, how would you feel?

Dejected and insecure, you wouldn't be able to see your partner as your port in the storm, and that would prompt you to seek comfort elsewhere.

The same is true for you. If you have expressed your feelings to your partner and he has been supportive of you, stop and take some time to listen to him. He needs support and comfort from you too, and if you are not the one to give it to him, he will seek it elsewhere.

Communication is about **listening**. When someone feels truly heard, they tend to feel *empowered, loved, supported, and understood*. Feeling heard satisfies our need to externalize our ideas and emotions, self-expression; it helps make us aware because the listener acts as a mirror, allows our thoughts and feelings to come out, so we can become aware in turn. It makes us feel appreciated, important, and value our affirmations because the other person is there. We live in a fast-paced world where people rarely have time to sit down and reflect on their feelings, let alone listen to someone else's. The lack of listening during communication drives people apart and makes the relationship unstable. This is why it's critical to develop your listening skills if you want your partner to feel loved and cared for. But listening involves much more than hearing.

Hearing is not Listening! There's a big difference.

To hear you simply need to use your hearing; listening, on the other hand, means *"recognizing" the signals around you*, being receptive to your surroundings in all circumstances where it is crucial to be able to pick up on the nuances. Unlike hearing, listening involves the use of the intellect. *Listening is a will.*

To listen, it is essential to understand others' facts, opinions, and feelings, put yourself in the other person's shoes, and understand their point of view. Therefore, a good listener avoids interrupting and coming to hasty conclusions and asks questions to learn more about who is in front of him. A conversation based on active listening is similar to a tennis match, in which the opponents study each other to understand each other's moves and hit the ball at the right moment. To listen is to perceive. There are different modes of listening:

- **PASSIVE**: this is a type of ineffective listening that takes place when words "go in one ear and out the other";

- **SELECTIVE**: is the one most commonly practiced when you hear only what you want to hear or, in other words, you filter the message;

- **REFLECTIVE**: allows you to act as a mirror and re-send to the speaker what he is saying, allowing him to acquire a new vision of what he has communicated verbally and non-verbally, helping to grasp new ideas, cope with dissatisfaction and problems of others without making judgments and reintegrating, if necessary, negative emotions;

- **ACTIVE**: it allows us to improve the ability to listen because it is feedback on what has been transmitted to us by our interlocutor. The listener gives back to the speaker what he or she has just heard, accompanying him or her in the exploration undertaken.

Selective listening, or pseudo-listening, is only partial listening to what the other person is saying, without paying much attention. This happens when:

- you start thinking about how to respond to what the other person is saying even before they have finished talking;

- you engage in other activities while the person in front of you is talking, such as looking at your phone.

Selectively listening to who is in front of us (even worse if it's our partner) can lead to many problems. People who have this habit have difficulty maintaining successful relationships precisely because they cannot fully process the information that other people share with them, which is very damaging in a relationship. Not feeling heard could also trigger feelings of anxiety in someone with fearful or worried attachment styles.

When your partner is talking to you, stop for a moment, put aside all distractions and listen to him, taking an interest in him. Don't interrupt him while he's talking by thinking about what you might say. Listen to him!

If you feel that your communication skills need some work and you want to improve your relationships, you need to learn how to actively listen to others. When you actively listen to your interlocutor, everything from your words, actions, and body language will show that you're paying attention. But what can you do to learn how to listen actively?

Here are some techniques that will help you focus your attention on the other person and make them feel heard without judging them:

ASKING QUESTIONS. Asking questions while the person in front of you is talking to you will help you stay focused on listening and better understand how the person speaking to you feels; moreover, the use of questions will help your interlocutor to gain clarity in his mind. Asking questions shows your sincere interest in the person who is talking to you;

it shows her that you are interested in what she is saying and you want to help her and be supportive.

PARAPHRASING. To paraphrase means to expound in your own words by developing or clarifying concepts expressed by someone. Doing this while listening to a person will help you to stay focused because you have to listen to what they are saying; repeating it in your own words will imprint it better in your mind and you will be sure that you understand what the person is saying and what their feelings are. Do not repeat "like a parrot" what the person has said. Try expressing it in your own words. This way you will focus on the message the person wants to convey to you.

Sometimes when someone is speaking, we can twist the message in our minds and interpret it in our way. Paraphrasing will also help us avoid this from happening. By rephrasing what your partner is saying to you, you will be able to understand their reasoning and you will have the confidence that you have heard them correctly.

By paying attention to the way he expresses what he is thinking, you will be able to empathize with his situation. If this behavior bothers him, explain that you are trying to listen carefully and put yourself in his shoes. As you get used to it, you will be able to do this mentally.

For example, if he has just told you that he has had a hellish day, you can tell him, *"You had a bad day at work because of your coworkers. Now you're feeling stressed and discouraged."* You can also use this method to clarify what he is saying. For example, you could reply like this, *"You would think you are angry at your boss because he talked to you in front of your other colleagues."*

The moment we say to the person in front of us, *"Let's see if I understand: ..."* or *"so you're telling me: ..."* and explain in our own words what we think we understand, we allow the listener to confirm or clarify misunderstandings. Doing this will allow both of us to be on the same page. You will put yourself in the speaker's shoes while the other person will feel understood and supported by you.

This is usually more than enough to show a person that you care about them. When someone talks to us about the problems, they just want to get out all the negative emotions they have inside that are weighing them down.

Sometimes though, on top of that, he *may* want some advice from us. Before giving ours, we should make sure that the person wants advice. Let's see what to do in this case.

FEEDBACK. After you have listened carefully to your interlocutor, asked questions to better understand what he is talking about, and expressed in your own words what he has tried to communicate to you, there is one more thing to do: you must provide feedback, that is, share your thoughts. When you give feedback to the person in front of you, you are showing that you have listened with interest to what they have told you and that you are interested.

In doing so, however, try to:

- **Be honest**: express what you think: don't tell the person "what they'd like to hear" if you know it won't help them resolve the situation;

- **Don't hurt the person in front of you**: being honest is fine but be careful *how* you say things. There are ways and ways to express what you think with respect and without hurting those on the other side;

- **Do not make judgments:** your purpose is to help the person in front of you and not to judge him. You may come to hasty conclusions and criticize his actions or state of mind if you judge him. In this case, you would not be a good listener. If you were in his situation, what would you want him to say to you? Would you want to be criticized and judged, or would you want practical help? Try to understand what he is saying or find out why he has behaved in a certain way.

  Be kind, express yourself in a calm tone, and don't be critical of him. Focus on his problem and put yourself in his shoes.

Your goal is not to determine whether he is wrong or right. You just need to try to see the situation from his perspective. Ask further questions to understand his position instead of judging him.

We've said it before, but we'll say it again.

Not everyone wants feedback while listening, so before you give advice, make sure your conversation partner does.

Talking to someone who listens to us using active listening makes us feel comfortable sharing even our deepest thoughts and emotions.

This is because the listener shows empathy without judging us and makes us feel understood and supported. Having this kind of conversation allows you to establish respect between people. If the person who actively listens to you is your partner, you will feel understood and safe, you will know that you can confide anything to him because he listens to you and tries to put himself in your shoes without judging himself.

Looking for solutions together brings you closer and makes your relationship grow constructively. Just as you're happy for your partner to listen to you when you're having problems or just a bad day, you should also strive to be supportive of him in the same way. If you don't think you're a good listener, but the tips we've offered into practice.

Active listening is a skill that can be acquired through awareness! Since we are not born with the predisposition to listen to others, but it is a skill that is acquired over time, you can acquire it too! Strive to be a good listener for your partner. Communication is the foundation of a relationship. Healthy communication will grow your relationship and decrease anxiety because you will both know you have a supportive and supportive partner!

Empathy in Relationships

As we have seen, to succeed in having good communication with your partner, you need to put in the effort. One quality that fosters communication is empathy. But what is empathy? And what does it entail?

The word empathy comes from the ancient Greek "εμπάθεια" *(empátheia),* a word composed of *en-* which means "within" and *pathos* which means "suffering or feeling". Therefore, empathy is the ability to make one's own the suffering of others, put oneself in their shoes, and place oneself immediately in the state of mind or situation of another person.

At the neurobiological level, the understanding of another person's mind and experiences is supported by a particular class of neurons: mirror neurons. Participating as witnesses to actions, sensations, and emotions of other individuals activates the same brain areas that are usually involved in performing the same actions and perceiving the same sensations and emotions.

This means that empathy is a skill that *allows us to recognize others' feelings and emotions as if they were our own* and thus allows us to understand the views and reactions of others.

An empathetic person offers his or her attention to another person by putting aside personal concerns and thoughts; he or she empathizes with their moods and thoughts. To show empathy towards someone, it is unnecessary to use words as this quality can also be expressed through body language.

However, putting oneself in someone's shoes does not mean agreeing with what they think, going along with them, and justifying them if they are wrong, or sharing a state of mind. The meaning of empathy is much deeper than that. You can show empathy towards someone even if you don't agree with their thoughts.

Showing empathy towards someone is like building a bridge between you and the other person. This invisible bridge allows you to tiptoe into the other person's world, stay there for the time necessary to understand the motivations and intensity of their emotional experience, and then return to be yourself, consistent with your existential reality.

Empathy is the basic element of human relationships because it facilitates interaction and mutual understanding. Understanding and sharing joy, pain, and a moment of anger with others are very important to maintain our interpersonal relationships.

Like all human characteristics, empathy can be more or less developed in various individuals for various reasons, such as their attachment style, constitutional predispositions, the influence of experience, and educational context. In short, some are more predisposed to be activated by the emotions of others and those who are less, but this depends a lot on how we have been accustomed in childhood and subsequent experiences to give attention or not to the emotional states of others.

It is important to know that many relationships, sentimental or otherwise, can have negative backlashes when empathy is lacking.

It is very difficult for a person who does not feel emotionally understood by their partner to be satisfied with the current relationship and continue to invest time and energy into it. In the worst-case scenario, this can lead to the decision to end the relationship. Therefore, if you want to improve your relationship, you need to be empathetic to your partner.

Do you feel that you are not very empathetic? We mentioned that empathy is a critically important social skill, and like all skills, it can be acquired. How to do it?

Empathy represents one of the basic tools of truly effective and rewarding interpersonal communication. The best thing you can do to foster mutual empathy within a relationship is to actively listen to the other person. You don't have to pay attention to just your words. Get out of your mindset, disregard your interests but consider those of your partner.

Listen carefully, ask questions to make sure you understand and don't make judgments about them. Showing empathy will allow you to access the feelings, moods. More generally, the whole world of your partner, learning also to understand what he wants to communicate through body language (posture, gestures, muscle tension, proxemics, facial expressions, tone, timbre and volume of voice, length of pauses, etc., say a lot about a person).

Therefore, we can consider empathy as a strategic form of communication, a sophisticated tool of emotional resonance, a kind of "emotional radar" with which to pick up and decode the weak signals of the mind and heart, the deepest moods, and hidden thoughts.

Empathy can bring two interlocutors closer together and produce positive effects on the level of mutual understanding.

When you show empathy towards your partner, you focus on him, understand him without judging him, or let your feelings take over. By putting yourself in his shoes, you can imagine his experiences and look at the situation from his point of view. Doing this is very important because it can lead you to improve your listening skills, make couple communication more effective, and create a deeper bond.

Nurturing empathy as a couple requires commitment and effort from both partners. Here are four areas you can work on or improve together:

- **SHARE HOW YOU FEEL.** To succeed in increasing empathy, it is important not only that you learn to listen to your partner, but also that you open up to them. It's not easy to talk about your feelings, but this way you can improve your relationship and build a deeper bond. Mutual empathy is nurtured by taking on the other person's feelings and communicating your own emotions. You can try saying, *"I'm feeling sad today"* or *"I enjoyed being with you."*

- **TALK ABOUT THE IMPORTANT THINGS.** Caught up in the usual routine, it can sometimes happen that you always talk about the same topics at the expense of deeper and more meaningful ones. Try to nurture empathy as a couple by bringing conversations to more important issues. For example, you can talk about your goals, dreams, desires, interests, and fears. Try addressing one of these topics every week or every day.

- By doing this, you can rediscover your dreams and hopes for the future.

  In these moments, avoid talking about household chores, children, work, or groceries. For example, you might say, *"Remember when you used to dream of traveling the world and seeing new places all the time? Lately, you haven't been talking about what you hope to do and achieve in life. Is that still your dream or do you have other desires?".*

- **PUT YOURSELF IN THEIR SHOES.** Many people confuse empathy with sympathy, and instead of putting themselves in the other person's shoes by empathizing with their situations, they show them sympathy.

Having feelings of pity or tenderness does not help you discuss your partner's feelings; on the contrary, in this way, there is a risk of imposing your feelings on the other person and not fully understanding their state of mind. Instead of saying, *"I know how you feel. I felt it too,"* and go on and on about your experience, try to respond empathetically, *"It must have been awful. I also felt something similar and I felt terrible. How do you feel after what happened?"* This type of communication encourages the other person to speak up and open up instead of closing themselves off from the other person's words.

- **BE OPEN**. When interacting and talking with your partner, do so openly, without closing yourself off mentally or physically. This will allow you to stay focused on your relationship, improve couple communication and build a deeper bond.

  Being open means *listening to your partner* and reflecting from **his** point of view. As you do this, strive to keep your body facing his direction by assuming a relaxed posture, avoiding moving away from him, crossing your arms, looking at your fingernails or phone, or leaving the room while talking. If you are both open and focused on your relationship, you will not pull away or create gaps and conflict between you.

We've seen how to successfully acquire this communication skill.

However, if you know that you have already acquired the ability to show empathy towards others, particularly your partner, you can still strive to improve it. How?

- **SEEK PHYSICAL CONTACT WITH YOUR PARTNER.** Demonstrations of affection help to create empathy in the relationship. Hug him, kiss him, hold his hand: these are simple and effective gestures that allow you to pay attention to your partner and establish a certain physical intimacy with him. Physical contact allows the body to produce oxytocin, a chemical that helps increase the feeling of happiness and reduces anxiety levels.

- **OBSERVE YOUR PARTNER.** You can develop more empathy for your partner by observing them. Imagine the thoughts that might be grazing his or her mind. See how he moves and pay attention to his body language.

  Body language can tell us a lot about a person. It can help you understand what he is feeling: *Is he nervous? Is he happy?*

  As you observe him, assimilate all the information you're getting and then see if his mood depends on a certain situation or what he's doing.

- **IMAGINE THINGS FROM HIS POINT OF VIEW.** Empathy is a very useful quality for resolving conflicts and differences because it allows you to understand what the other person is thinking. Instead of reacting impulsively, stop for a moment. Close your eyes and put yourself in your partner's shoes. Think about how he or she sees the situation or interprets your behaviors. As you do this, consider some aspects of his past, such as his relationship with his parents, other family members, his worldview, and so on.

- With this information, you will have the opportunity to better understand his decisions, behaviors, and how certain events have affected him.

  When trying to empathize with your partner, don't think about what you would have done in his or her place - that's not the goal of empathy. Rather, consider everything you know about him and his past and understand the extent to which these aspects led him to take on a certain reaction. If you think that your partner's reaction to an event is exaggerated, look at things from his perspective; consider his attachment style and past experiences. By analyzing the situation in this way, you will be able to put yourself in the other person's shoes and perhaps their reaction will seem tolerable.

  If you both can take this attitude, instead of fighting, you will be able to deal with the problem and each of you will be able to see it from the other's point of view.

- **DO ACTIVITIES FOR A COUPLE.** Good exercises to foster couple empathy include acting, role-playing, and imitation. Why not try taking a dance class for couples? Engaging in these activities together allows you to learn more about your partner, increase empathy in your relationship, strengthen your bond and see things from his or her point of view.

Therefore, we can conclude that empathy is a cognitive process, a skill that can be practiced, trained, and in which you can become an expert. As you strive to acquire this skill or improve it within your relationship, try to be flexible in deciding when, how, and how much to activate the empathic feeling.

Based on the intensity of empathy we demonstrate towards others, we can distinguish different types:

- **Affective**: it concerns our ability to feel emotions, sensations, and feelings experienced by someone else and feel compassion for this person; in a nutshell: *"I feel what you feel"*;

- **Cognitive**: it is the ability that allows us to have more complete and precise knowledge about the contents of the mind of the person in front of us; in a nutshell: *"I understand what is happening to you"*;

- **Excess empathy or "hyper-empathy"**: it is a kind of mirror and sponge. Not only do we feel what others feel, but we suffer it ourselves and it is physical pain and one that subjects us to the needs of others, without being able to distinguish this boundary between us and others.

Just as the absence of empathy for others, especially our partner, can cause serious damage within a relationship, the same can be said of excess empathy. In both cases, both the absence and **excess of empathy** can cause nervous breakdowns and depression. If you find yourself in one of these extremes, you certainly can't be in a position to help others.

A person who can't handle empathy can end up getting lost in the needs of others, "poisoning" themselves through excessive compassion to the point of feeling guilty about the pain others experience. This can become exhausting in the long run.

An example of excess empathy can be seen in women who can understand their partners' psychopathic behavior and even justify it. Their excess of empathy makes them completely *unable to see* the predator, killer, or tormentor in front of them, and as a result, they justify their partner's acts of violence.

As always in life, excesses are not good and the ideal is always to have a certain **balance**. It is also important to have balance as you acquire the ability to put yourself in the shoes of others. As you learn to do this, don't confuse "yourself" with the "self" of others. It is true that *"empathy is the ability to put ourselves in the shoes of those in front of us," but at the same time it is important "not to forget to be yourself".*

Create Trust in the Couple

Trust is the foundation of free, uninhibited, generous, and authentic love.

Trust is the starting point of a relationship, that is, the basis on which to build and strengthen it. Trust has the power to make each partner feel heard, supported, and be themselves without fear of the other's judgment. Trusting someone means *"trusting and giving oneself in a relationship with the knowledge that the other can welcome, support, and protect."*

The happiest and most fulfilling relationships are built on a very solid foundation of unconditional trust. To get the most out of your relationship, both you and your partner must learn to create such trust.

Many people believe that trust is solely about sexual fidelity, but while this is an important aspect, a trust includes so many other aspects. Here are some things you can do to **build trust** in your relationship:

LOVE SINCERELY. Both of you need to know that you are loved for the people you are and not for any other reasons, such as money, family, physical appearance, or even fear of being alone. Sincerely love your partner for who they are and make sure your relationship is based on love.

BE FAITHFUL. Lack of fidelity is one of the leading causes of anxiety in romantic relationships and separation. If one of the two is unfaithful, it is as if he destroys "the bricks" that put the basis of building his relationship. Sometimes people can overcome a betrayal, but it is very difficult to do so. Being faithful to a person means being faithful on all levels, not only sexually but also emotionally. Some people believe that establishing an intimate bond with someone other than your partner, just spending time together, is not harmful to the couple, but it is not true.

It's time you're taking away from your partner to devote to another person, and over time your relationship suffers.

RESPECT YOUR PARTNER. Trust only develops in healthy and safe environments. If you and your partner attack each other verbally or physically or reject each other, it only triggers unnecessary fears that can jeopardize your relationship's trust. Strive to remain calm in any situation. Remember the basic rules we saw at the beginning of the chapter?

Keeping a calm tone of voice will help you with this. Don't try to control your partner's every move, but respect their space. If your partner wants to spend time with friends, try to show agreement but make it clear upfront what behaviors are acceptable and what are not. For example, if one of you wants to go clubbing with friends but the other has concerns about it, talk about it in advance so that you can prevent any problems or bad feelings in the future.

Giving your partner space to himself allows him to reflect on how much he misses you and how much he appreciates your company. In other words, this way you offer the other person the opportunity to approach you of their own free will, and this is a great way to build connection and trust.

TALK ABOUT YOUR NEEDS. When you and your partner clearly explain what your needs are and look for common ground with each other, you become stronger and nurture trust in your relationship.

TALK ABOUT UNCOMFORTABLE TOPICS. There are many "uncomfortable" topics that people tend not to bring up in a relationship for fear that they might create tension. One such topic, for example, is "money." Money has to do with freedom and security, both of which are fundamental aspects of life. Not addressing this topic is letting a lurking danger get in the way of your trust in the relationship at any time. If you and your partner have similar views about money, it's much easier to act in harmony, like a team achieving the same goal.

COMPARE YOUR SCALES OF VALUES. During the getting-to-know-you phase, you have already learned a lot about your partner.

However, you may not have paused to compare the priorities in life for each of you. Talk about it and try to figure out if you are building your lives and expectations on the same values or if you share values that will determine your choices throughout life.

Even if you have different values, the important thing is to get to know each other well so that you can better understand your partner's intuitive processes and the way they tend to judge situations.

SPEND QUALITY TIME TOGETHER. Spending quality time with your partner is not about eating dinner together in front of the TV every night; it is about feeling connected, exchanging feelings, and appreciating each other's company. Spending quality time together awakens curiosity and excitement about the other person, which deepens the feeling of connection and trust in your relationship. Try turning off your phone when you're spending time with your partner and devote yourself only to them.

MAKE YOUR RELATIONSHIP YOUR PRIORITY. Taking the other person's presence for granted and neglecting them is very easy. Try not to use up all your energy interacting with other people or going about your daily activities. If living a happy relationship is one of your main life goals, make sure that your partner always remains at the top of your priority list. Every once in a while, stop and take some time to reflect on what you value most in your partner and what they give or do for you.

In our fast-paced world, it's easier to notice what your partner doesn't do, what they could do better, or what they've done wrong than it is to appreciate what they do every day. So make sure you give enough attention to what works between you or what your partner does well and let them know.

Mutual gratitude generates feelings of trust and admiration in the couple.

OVERCOME DIFFICULTIES. Misunderstandings, fights, and arguments can happen. Make sure that a normal disagreement or outburst of anger doesn't force your partner to fear being abandoned. If you reassure your partner and overcome difficulties together, confidence in your relationship will increase.

Every relationship brings problems and adversity, but trust grows and becomes more solid every day when difficulties are faced with an open mind. We've seen how you can create you can build trust within your relationship. Now we'll look at how you can increase the trust you have in your partner. There are several ways to do this. Below are a few of them:

1. **Believe in his abilities**: if you think that your partner is not able to do something, you are showing that you do not have confidence in him. Talk about it calmly, and together you can find a constructive solution so you can keep your mutual trust solid;

2. **Trust:** if you want your partner to trust you, you have to show that you trust him/her. Only by demonstrating mutual trust can you have a successful relationship.

Often the presence of trust is linked to our inner feelings. If you have realized that you have an insecure attachment style throughout these chapters, your insecurity could jeopardize the strength of your relationship. To have a stable relationship and grow the trust you have in your partner, you will have to learn to put your vulnerability aside. Unless some facts prove otherwise, you have to trust the person you love. Give them the benefit of the doubt. Your insecurity and lack of trust in others can lead you to always expect the worst to happen in every situation. For example, if you call your partner but he doesn't answer, you may think he is cheating on you because of your insecurity. Just because he didn't call you doesn't mean he is cheating on you. Having trust in a person means always being willing to give them the benefit of the doubt. Don't jump to conclusions! Always give your partner a chance to explain themselves before concluding;

3. **Don't touch his or her phone**: have you both set a password to access your phone? If the answer is yes, you may have trouble trusting each other. When trust is real, both partners respect each other's privacy while having unfettered access to each other's information. If you think the person who is calling your partner may be a threat to your relationship, it means you have a serious trust issue and you need to address it;

4. **Let him/her off the hook:** when trust is lacking, you feel the need to monitor each other's every step, always know what he/she is doing and who he/she is with. If you don't trust your partner, you may feel threatened by anyone who comes near him and you may become extremely possessive.

134

Trust is based on fully relying on the other person by allowing them to act freely;

this will also boost your self-esteem and help you grow your relationship in a healthy way.

In addition to creating and growing trust within a relationship, it is very important **to show** your partner that they enjoy your trust. How can you go about showing them?

1. **Maintain your routine.** Many people try to continually plan something new to surprise each other because they believe it allows them to have a fabulous relationship. It's nice to surprise each other from time to time, but a solid relationship isn't just about that. For a relationship to be *long-lasting,* it is necessary to have stability and also repetitiveness. That last word might give the idea of boredom and monotony, but for things to work in the long run, you need to be predictable. Would you feel secure in a relationship where you never know what to expect each day? No, that's because trust is based on predictability.

2. **Be reliable**. You are confident that you can always count on your partner when you know their behaviors and reactions, regardless of the circumstances. Knowing that you can always count on someone in any situation gives you a feeling of security. Do the same thing with your partner so that he/she can always count on you. Be consistent! Consistency is one of the key factors of trust.

For example, if you said you will be home by 7 pm, try to be on time and remember to let your partner know in case you have something unexpected and are forced to arrive late.

If 4 times out of 5 you're going to be late without even bothering to give notice, you'll show that your needs far outweigh your partner's and that your relationship isn't the most important thing to you. To have a happy relationship, you must both strive to be reliable and consistent. If you do this, you will decrease the stress and anxiety within your relationship because you will have the confidence that each one is doing their best to keep their commitments while always taking into account the needs of the other.

3. **Be honest**. With time, you will surely have acquired the ability to understand if your partner lies, if he tries to hide something from you, or if he avoids telling you what he thinks. Know that your partner also has the same ability. So, when you lie, hide things, or don't say what you think, your partner might notice and feel betrayed. On top of that, you demolish your relationship's trust because you show that you don't trust him and create anxiety within your relationship. Secrets are landmines within a relationship; at any moment they can explode and bring out the truth with its consequences. Knowing that you can blindly trust your partner's words and that each person is committed to expressing their thoughts to the other in a kind way allows you to build a strong bond.

Remember that your partner isn't a fortune teller and can't even read your mind, so if there's something that's bothering you, talk openly with him or her about it without expecting him or her to guess it. You'll avoid unnecessary tension, stress, and anxiety from building up and you'll calmly resolve the issue together as a real team!

4. **Learn to say no**. Paying attention to your partner's needs and trying to meet them is certainly correct, but sometimes it's important to know how to say no. It's not possible to do everything all the time, and the occasional refusal will only increase their respect for you. In the long run, taking a stand and imposing yourself *when the need arises* will help increase mutual trust in your relationship.

In a couple's relationship, it is normal to have problems, doubts, and misunderstandings, yet if you both believe in your relationship, and can do a lot to increase mutual trust and make your relationship even stronger. It is essential that you show each other respect and trust, otherwise you can risk ruining your story deep down. Having trust in someone is not easy, it is hard work, especially when you experience moments when you feel betrayed, abandoned, and not understood by those who tell us they love us. Building a solid relationship based on mutual trust takes a long time; losing trust, on the other hand, only takes a moment. If your partner loses trust in you, it will be very difficult for you to regain it.

Lack of trust in love can depend on several causes, which have to do with the dynamics of the couple and the vision and consideration you have of yourself. Trust cannot exist when you go behind your partner's back (for example, by cheating on them).

Once trust is destroyed, it can no longer be fully restored because it will always be undermined by doubt. Let's see what are some of the causes that can lead you to lose trust in your partner and what you can do to recover trust.

- **BETRAYAL.** This is one of the main causes that create a difficult wound for those who have been betrayed. Even when the infidelity seems to overcome, it is very difficult to completely recover the partner's trust because he will continue to live with the fear of being betrayed again.

- **LOW SELF-ESTEEM.** A person with an insecure attachment style may harbor unconscious thoughts that they do not deserve their partner's love and affection. This feeling can manifest itself in the form of control and mistrust and hurts the relationship; your partner will think they can never earn your trust, making your relationship unstable. In this case, we recommend that you see a specialist so you can address the causes of your low self-esteem.

- **INABILITY TO TRUST.** If you lived a childhood with traumatic abandonment experiences and separations, this can affect your relationship in a negative way; your brain will always activate a self-defense mechanism that will prevent you from trusting your partner completely. You will not be able to have true intimacy with your partner because you will always be afraid of being hurt. Again, we recommend that you consult a specialist. He will help you to identify the causes of your inability to trust people and overcome them. Doing this will help you to have a healthy and lasting reaction.

- **DIFFERENT EXPECTATIONS.** We've talked a lot about the importance of communication.

If you and your partner don't communicate from the beginning of your relationship about what your goals and values are important to you, you may find out too late that you have different life expectations. Talk about uncomfortable topics, your dreams, travel, the future together, etc., early on. If you don't, you may find yourself in destabilizing and frustrating situations, for one or both of you, that undermine trust and feelings in the long run.

- **SEXUAL PROBLEMS.** Sex is fundamental to a couple, and if problems in this area are not addressed, it is easy for one partner to interpret this as a lack of desire for him or, worse, as a desire for someone else. It is important to talk about this openly. If you do, you will avoid increasing anxiety and stress in your relationship and show that you trust your partner.

- **LACK OF COMMUNICATION.** If you fail to have good communication and realize that it's more the things you don't say than the things you do say, some distance may arise between you. Mutual silences only increase the already existing distance and this can cause misunderstandings and distrust to arise in your relationship that undermines your bond.

- **JEALOUSY.** Feelings of possession, constant questions, interrogations, assumptions, frequent tantrums, if not kept at bay, can destroy trust (especially in those who suffer it) and make your partner run away.

- **LIE.** Whether they're big, small, or "for good," all lies tarnish your relationship to the point of making esteem and trust truly impossible.

When you lose trust in the person you love, it can set off a chain reaction of other problems that go on to wear down the relationship, even to the point of questioning everything. Feeling that you can no longer count on your partner's support can lead to feeling annoyed at everything they do, losing respect, and pulling out aggression. As a result, endless arguments will arise where you seek conflict and not resolution because you accuse each other. Over time, this situation can create great emotional exhaustion, depression, and communication problems, which can even lead to the breakup of the relationship if not addressed. This whole whirlwind of problems is caused by one thing: lack of trust.

The best way to get out of it is to quickly and sincerely recognize that something is not working, name the emotions you are feeling, and dare to communicate them first to yourself and then to the other person. In this way, you will be able to reopen a path of communication open to dialogue and confrontation. How can you win back your partner's trust? Here are some exercises that will help you regain trust in love.

1. **Learn to communicate at the right time.** It takes time to be able to restore a good dialogue or learn how to do it. It is necessary to look at each other unhurriedly and tell each other's needs and desires.

2. **Train trust.** You can do some fun little exercises as a couple that help activate the ability to rely on the other person to feel supported and welcomed.

For example, you can ask your partner to fall backward and reassure them that you will be behind them to catch and support them; or you can blindfold them and tell them to let you guide them. You can sit across from each other, looking into each other's eyes, hands in hands, and tell each other, "I trust you trust me." These small exercises can develop your personal ability to trust and ask for trust.

3. **Forgive**. If wounds from the past have not healed, it is necessary to work on forgiveness and the reasons that caused rifts in your relationship.

4. **Distinguish your problems from those of the couple.** One of you may have old wounds from your childhood. It is important to recognize which behaviors are related to past traumas and which are related to the couple's dynamics. If you can distinguish between these two types of problems, you won't be dumping frustrations, anger, and emotions on your partner, for which they are not to blame.

As we said at the beginning of this consideration of trust, this quality is easy to acquire but very difficult to recover. We have tried to encapsulate in a few pages good advice to **create** trust within a relationship, **increase** trust in your partner, **show him** in practical ways that he has your trust **to recover** it if it has been "destroyed". Sometimes, however, even applying all these tips, you can no longer trust your partner.

In this case, learn to understand when it's time to walk away. If you stay in an unhappy and painful relationship for too long, it will increase your insecurity and decrease your self-confidence.

This will make it harder for you to believe in another relationship that might be right for you. This is why you must be honest with yourself about how much trust you can place in the other person. Of course, we hope that all the tips and advice in this manual will help you improve or save your relationship.

Learn to Forgive and Apologize

Forgiveness. Usually, this word makes us think of the moment when we accept someone's apology. But to fully understand the meaning of this word, let's go back to its etymology for a moment. **Forgiveness** comes from Medieval Latin and is a word composed of *"per,"* a prefix of completely, and *"to give."* So to forgive means *to give completely.* When the Latin "forgive" was adopted into the Germanic ancestor of English, it was translated piece by piece, making the result what linguists call a *"calque"* (from the French *"calquer,"* to trace or copy) literal transliteration. "For" was replaced by *"for,"* a prefix meaning "completely" in this case, and "donate" with *"giefan"* ("to give"). The result, *"forgeiefan,"* appeared in Old English meaning *"surrender, allow, "forgive for an offense," "give up anger against someone."*

Forgiving someone who has hurt or betrayed you is not always easy, it is one of the most difficult things to do in the course of life.

However, if you are planning to rebuild your relationship with someone, or if you simply want to put the past behind you and look forward, learning to forgive is essential.

To be able to forgive someone who has hurt you, it is first necessary for you to deal with your negative emotions and confront the person who has hurt you. In the long run, anger could become harmful. Forgiving someone who has hurt you can be very difficult indeed, and, naturally, your first reaction will be to hold a grudge and blame the person who has hurt you. Know, however, that letting anger and hurt dominate your thoughts will hurt you far more than it will hurt the person your resentment is directed at. Holding a grudge can ruin your future relationships with other people, cause you to become anxious and depressed, make you live in resentment, and isolate you from others. When you choose to forgive, not only can you rebuild your relationship with those who have hurt you, but you will primarily be doing good for yourself.

Forgiving is a **choice** and when you make it, you make a conscious decision to let go of negativity and move on. We know that forgiving is not an easy decision, much less a spontaneous one. To get to the point of deciding to forgive someone who has hurt you, you have to commit. It is not a spontaneous or simple act. Forgiveness is something you have to work at, but by choosing to forgive those who have hurt you, the person who will benefit the most from this decision will be you. If you choose to forgive your partner, there are two things you need to do:

1. Deal with the negative emotions;

2. Confront the person who hurt you.

Let's first look at how you can deal with negative emotions.

REMOVE NEGATIVE EMOTIONS. Detach yourself from any negative feelings you have about the other person. Try crying, engaging in intense physical activity, going to a secluded place and screaming, or anything else that allows you to release all of your hurt. This will help you heal your wounds and move on. If you don't throw out all the negative emotions, they will become more intense and cause you to suffer even more. You must learn to trust yourself again, your judgment, and your ability to make informed decisions. Subsequently, you can begin to recover it about the other person.

BROADEN YOUR POINT OF VIEW. Take a step back and look at the situation more objectively. Did your partner intentionally hurt you? Did he realize he had hurt you? Did he or she try to apologize and make things right with you? Reconsider everything and calmly analyze the situation: if you can understand how and why it came about, it will be easier for you to forgive. Then, ask yourself honestly how many times you have done wrong to him and others (even if you didn't want to) and how many times he or they have forgiven you. Remember how you felt and the relief and gratitude you felt when you are the one receiving forgiveness. We all make mistakes. People hurt us even unintentionally, but remember that we do it to them too, and thinking about how we feel when that happens allows us to look at things more objectively.

TALK TO SOMEONE. If at this point you still haven't been able to forgive your partner or anyone who has wronged you, and you feel you still have feelings of anger and frustration, talk to someone. Confiding in someone you trust will help you process your feelings and gain an unbiased point of view.

Talk to a friend, family member, or therapist, someone who can listen or perhaps offer you a shoulder to cry on. The very fact that you are venting to someone outside the situation may help get a big weight off your chest.

EXPRESS POSITIVE EMOTIONS. By getting to this point you should have removed some of your negative emotions. Finding a way to express positive emotions will help you release negative and destructive feelings and overcome your problems. For example, you can keep a journal, write letters, paint, dance, listen to music. Keep your mind busy by doing what makes you happy, helps you eliminate tension, and makes you feel good. Making room for positive emotions will make you more aware of the problems you face and allow you to recognize and master negative feelings instead of ignoring them.

TIME. Although forgiving is a choice, you can't forgive a person the instant you choose to. It takes self-control, determination, compassion, and most importantly, time. There is no ideal time frame for maturing forgiveness. You may find yourself holding a grudge for days, months, or even years before you realize that you can't help but reconcile with the other party. Remember that the really important things in life are love, empathy, and forgiveness and that no one has ever come to the end of their life thinking, *"I should have held anger for longer."* Even if it takes time to get there, forgiving is always the best choice you can make.

Forgiving someone does not mean allowing the other person to continue to be a part of your life. Maybe your forgiveness won't mean anything to the person you've given so much to. Sometimes it is not possible at all to rebuild a relationship.

145

However, even if the situation didn't work out as you hoped, you did the right thing. Forgiving is a noble action and you will not regret doing it.

Even if you forgive your partner, you can decide if you intend to mend the relationship with him/her or let him/her go. Before making this decision, you need to think long and deeply about your relationship. Is it worth rebuilding it? Is there a chance that he/she will hurt you one more time if you let him/her get close again? In some situations, such as in abusive relationships or if your partner cheats on you several times, it is healthier and safer to exclude him from your life. You deserve better. However, if you've decided to forgive, you need to forget the past and focus on the future. If you feel that the relationship is worth rebuilding, then you can slowly start moving forward. Tell the other person that you still love them despite their betrayal and want them to be a part of your life.

If you keep digging through the wounds of the past, you will never be able to truly forget and move on. Look for the bright side and see the situation as an opportunity to start over and make your relationship stronger and more solid.

By getting to this point, you've managed to deal with your negative emotions. All that's left is for you to confront the person who hurt you. Let's see how you can do that.

DON'T MAKE HASTY JUDGMENTS. Don't make hasty judgments about the person who has hurt you; you may say or do things that you will regret later.

Before you act, take some time to deal well with your emotions and see things objectively. Before you say something you might regret or before you permanently eliminate this person from your life, think about everything you've experienced together and calmly and rationally assess whether this is an isolated offense or a repeated attitude.

LISTEN. Ask your partner or the person who hurt you to meet in a quiet, uncrowded place. Broaching the subject doesn't necessarily mean that things will go back to exactly the way they were between you, but listening to her side of the story will help you see things from her perspective before making a decision. As you listen to her, apply the communication, listening, and empathy techniques that you learned in this chapter. Try to stay calm and let her talk without interrupting or contradicting her.

SHOW COMPASSION. Try to put yourself for a moment in the shoes of the person who has hurt you. Imagine yourself in her place. Ask yourself, what would I have done in a similar situation? Would I have behaved differently? Try to understand what her reasons or intentions were. Did she intentionally want to hurt you? Did she have your best interests at heart? Or did she just act superficially?

DON'T ATTACK HIM. When confronting the person who has hurt you, make an effort to remain calm. Don't attack them in anger or hurl accusations or insults at them. You might regret it soon after, but in the meantime permanently ruin your relationship.

Instead of having an accusatory tone and saying, *"You made me feel like ..."*, *try saying, "I feel like ...".* Breathe deeply, stay calm, and don't respond if you are accused.

COMMUNICATE YOUR FEELINGS. Explain in a clear, calm, and balanced way how much he hurt you and how his behavior made you feel. If you don't, anger and resentment are likely to settle in, making sincere forgiveness impossible. Clarify how all of this has affected your relationship. Then look ahead. If you've decided to forgive your partner for his or her behavior, don't dwell on this episode and how it hurt you every time you argue. If you've decided to forgive, it's time to look forward.

DON'T RETALIATE. If you're trying to forgive your partner, you must abandon the idea of "getting even" or getting revenge. For example, if your partner cheated on you, you won't solve anything by getting even; in fact, you'll only cause more pain and resentment. Your forgiveness is worthless if you only grant it after you get your revenge, plus you will hurt more people, including yourself. Strive to show a more mature attitude by committing to regaining trust in your relationship. In this chapter, we have seen many ways you can do this.

TURN THE PAGE. Not everyone can apologize. If the person who hurt you asks for forgiveness, he or she will feel grateful and relieved at the thought that you can commit to rebuilding the relationship. If, on the other hand, he doesn't ask for it, by forgiving him you will have gotten a weight off your chest and can move on with your life. When you forgive someone, you prevent negative feelings from consuming you psychologically and physically.

When you decide to forgive yourself, throw out all the negative emotions, and focus on the positive, which makes you feel at peace with yourself.

This does not mean that things between you and the person who hurt you will go back to the way they were. If you feel that you can no longer trust the other person because they have hurt you too many times, that's still okay. The important thing is that you are clear with him or her.

But what if you are the one who has hurt your partner?

In this case, it is important to be able to pronounce a magic word composed of 5 letters: "EXCUSE".

Apologizing means *admitting that you have made a mistake*, that you are prone to the possibility of error; it means *admitting that you are responsible for your actions*. You are aware that we can harm someone by making a mistake else. Simply put, when you apologize you are admitting that you are human.

Since we live in a society that seems to value the strongest, the bully, those who prevaricate, mock, those who are unscrupulous and uncaring, for many, this little word weighs more than a boulder. Not everyone can admit to being wrong. For many, to apologize is to be weak, incapable, saying "excuse me" they pass as fools, losers, and not very confident.

Contrary to what many people think, apologizing is not an act of weakness but a strength. Only those who are confident are not afraid to admit that they may be wrong.

To apologize, it is necessary to be aware of what we are doing and the people we may be hurting.

Knowing how to apologize is not an innate skill, on the contrary, it is something that is learned. Perhaps when you were a child, your parents forced you to apologize to the friend you had shoved on some occasions.

Being able to apologize is very important in a relationship. Saying *"I'm sorry, I was wrong"*, *"I know I hurt you"*, *"I'm sorry I hurt you"* means gaining awareness and moving on without holding grudges. Simply saying "please forgive me" is not the same as saying sorry. You haven't even admitted that you were wrong! Show yourself truly sorry for what you did and show your partner that you want to make up for your mistake. If you have apologized:

- Be sincere when you apologize. Don't be irritated, otherwise, your partner will think that you are apologizing only out of a sense of duty and not because you are sincerely sorry;

- Take responsibility for your mistakes*: "I'm sorry I offended you."* Don't say, "I'm sorry you were offended" or "I'm sorry for the things that offended you" - these aren't real apologies; you're not admitting any responsibility for the situation. The only message you're sending is that you think it's the other person's fault for being offended too easily;

- Don't try to get the other person to forgive you by playing on your guilt, loneliness, or anxiety of waiting, and don't constantly ask if they are still angry with you. This will make you seem impatient and selfish. We have seen that forgiveness takes time, so be patient;

- Don't judge yourself if your partner eventually accepts your apology, don't conclude with more justifications. You will make the atmosphere tense again. Suggest spending time alone with your partner by going to lunch together or involving them in activities that allow you to reopen the bridge of communication.

If, on the other hand, your partner does not accept your apology or needs a greater amount of time to accept it, thank them for listening to you and leave open the possibility of future reconciliation. You might say, *"I understand that you are still angry with me, but thank you for allowing me to apologize. If you change your mind, call me."*

Resolving Conflict and How to Save a Relationship

Regardless of how compatible or deeply in love you and your partner are, you will have some clashes sooner or later. When two people spend a lot of their time together, it's normal for disagreements to arise. When you find yourself facing an argument, don't immediately think of it as a wake-up call. Very often, as a result of an exchange of opinions, you can have an even stronger bond with your partner. Therefore, there is no need to avoid conflicts that may arise between you and your partner, but you must learn how to manage them.

In this chapter, we have looked at many aspects that can help you save your relationship.

First and foremost, you need to set goals in your relationship, learn to communicate using various communication techniques and active listening, show empathy for each other, commit to growing trust within your relationship and know how to apologize and forgive each other. These are the foundations for having a successful relationship.

To smooth out a relationship problem, the first thing you need to do is accept your share of responsibility. Ask yourself, *"What am I currently doing to make my relationship situation worse?"* Instead of analyzing your partner's shortcomings, try reflecting on how your behavior helps perpetuate the problem. In fact, in some situations, we can decide to change the only thing that can be changed: ourselves.

If you are very angry, always give yourself time to stop and reflect on what you are saying. This will be helpful so that you don't say things you might regret just because you are in the grip of emotion. Try not to focus on thoughts of indignation, victimhood, or anger; rather, ask yourself, *"What is the real problem for me? What do I want? How can I look at the problem from my partner's perspective? What would my partner like? What can I do to make the problem worse? What, instead, to solve it? In what ways can I express myself more clearly?"* In this way you can attempt to reconnect with your spouse and speak with a different intent and greater awareness; it will also be easier to demonstrate empathy and put yourself in the other person's shoes. By doing this, you will no longer see your partner as a "criminal," but you will begin to think that they didn't have bad intentions.

For example, if your partner is doing his best to overcome a difficult situation at work and, due to fatigue, he burns dinner or ruins an object that you particularly care about, try to put yourself in his shoes. After all, his intent was, despite his fatigue, to do something for you. Would you still be upset knowing this?

Dialogue is always the best way to solve problems in a relationship. It is paradoxical because to have dialogue you need trust, but if this is lacking in the relationship, the only way to rebuild it is to dialogue. Dialogue means:

- **Exposing** calmly and a certain amount of affection, the reasons that led you to not trust your partner. By keeping calm and treating each other with respect, you will be able to have good communication. By doing this, you will be able to make your partner understand what the cause of your impatience is and how it made you feel. Remember not to attack him, not to accuse him by saying what he did or did not do;

- **Know how to listen** without preconceptions and taking time to reflect on your partner's words, without judging or labeling them. When there is love, dialogue strengthens the relationship and helps to find that drive to continue.

If dialogue is impossible or if the lack of trust fails, it's time to think about looking forward and moving on. Trust is something that a couple must work on their whole life if they want to move forward in a stable relationship. The first thing to do is to communicate healthily and effectively, so set aside time during the day to spend with your partner.

Talking and discussing problems will help you deal with them together. Each of you will be able to contribute to finding a solution.

If you hurt each other, be prepared to apologize, admit your part in the situation, and be ready to forgive. If wounds from the past have not healed, it is important to work on forgiveness. If it is necessary, see a specialist and pursue therapy to achieve safety.

One of the causes of lack of confidence in a relationship is lack of self-confidence and low self-esteem. If you are the one suffering from this, reflect and work on "self-knowledge" and, if necessary, consult a specialist.

Never forget that you and your partner are a team. Just as the two pilots mentioned at the beginning of the chapter need to support each other to reach the destination, in the same way, you and your partner need to work together on your relationship to achieve success. Lack of trust in the couple hinders the development of the relationship, while commitment, confidence, and sincerity are key to strengthening the bond and overcoming any difficult times together.

Remember that the little things count the most in a relationship and grow love, appreciation, and trust. Try giving a small kindness or a small surprise to your partner at a time when they are particularly tired and stressed. At times like these, it is essential to express words of reassurance, appreciation, and affection. It's much easier to accept someone's opinion when you feel that person cares about you and appreciates what you do.

By putting these little tips into practice, you will be able to make your bond stronger and create a great foundation for healthy communication. Communicating well in difficult situations is hard work, but you will find harmony and have a successful relationship if you work hard at it.

Chapter 5: What You Can Do to Combat Anxiety in Your Relationship

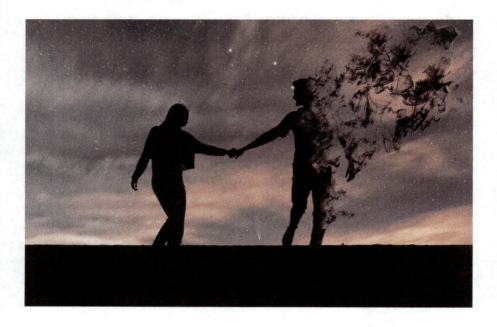

In a relationship, it is **crucial** to *openly share concerns* with your partner, especially if they generate feelings of withdrawal, isolation, or verbal attack on the other person. Make an effort to always express your feelings. Communicate. People who fail to express their feelings tend to be much more anxious, and this insecurity leads them to demand attention often. When you can't express how you feel, your anxiety tends to increase to the point where you can't manage your feelings and emotions; this leads to a defensive attitude.

It is also essential to find time to "decompress" some thoughts or fears that crowd the mind because they do nothing but drain time and energy (physical and mental). We live in a fast-paced world where anxiety and stress have become an integral part of it. Many may think that to combat anxiety, it is enough to avoid situations that cause stress; but getting rid of anxiety is not that simple! In cases where anxiety tends to be present in an excessive way, so much so that you can no longer control it, it is important to seek professional help so that you can find the root of your fears, understand them, deal with them in a safe environment, and develop effective coping strategies that will improve your health and your relationship.

In the previous chapter, we saw how anxiety creeps into relationships. Here are some practical things you can do if anxiety...

- **BREAKS TRUST.** Train your brain to live in the present. If you notice fear or worry that pulls your thoughts away from the facts of the present moment, pause and think about what you know (as opposed to what you don't know). Calm down before you act. Share openly when you feel worried and reach out to your partner (physically or verbally)

- **SQUASH YOUR TRUE VOICE.** Acknowledge your feelings sooner rather than later. A feeling or concern doesn't have to be a disaster to be addressed. Approach your partner with kindness and take your time to decompress some of the thoughts or fears circulating in your mind; they are draining your time and energy.

- **MAKES YOU BEHAVE SELFISHLY.** Take care of your needs, not your fears. When you notice yourself becoming fearful or overly defensive, take a moment to consider the compassion you have for yourself and your partner.

- **DEVELOP ACCEPTANCE.** Practice managing discomfort. There is no need to ignore or obsess over an uncomfortable thought. Take constructive action if you can. Sometimes your partner just needs you to be present with their feelings, and sometimes you need to offer yourself that same opportunity.

- **KIDNAP JOY.** Don't take yourself too seriously. You can use your sense of humor to overcome anxiety. Remember to laugh and play with your partner. Joy heals physically and comforts the brain in ways that are vital to a healthy relationship.

Increasing trust within your relationship reduces the power of anxiety. When you understand how anxiety affects your relationships, you may be able to make the appropriate changes to learn how to manage the stress and anxiety that comes with it. If you let negative thoughts and fears affect your relationship, you won't experience joy in your relationship and will put it at risk. However, by learning to manage stress and anxiety, you will have better sexuality and intimacy with your partner. As anxiety weakens, your relationship will grow stronger! If you and your partner can't overcome it, get help from an expert; this way you can get back to living peacefully and experiencing joy in your relationship.

The first thing you need to do to combat anxiety within your relationship is: **identify the root cause of your anxiety.** Why are you afraid that your partner doesn't like you enough? Why do you think you are not the right person for him/her? Why are you afraid that he/she will leave you? When you meet someone you like, and you want to develop a relationship with that person do you hide sides of yourself that you think they might not like? Do you pretend to be who you are not? Be honest!

As you continue in your relationship, bad memories from your past may resurface, which you're not proud of, which may make you feel unworthy of love. Don't let bad thoughts make their way into your mind! They could generate anxiety and stress. Face them. If there's something in your past that you're ashamed of, you can probably be terrified that your partner will find out. While you don't have to share every single aspect of your past with your partner, remember that keeping a big secret can create a lot of anxiety in your relationship. If you feel that you are understood and understood by your partner and your relationship of mutual trust is growing, talk to them. Share your concerns with your partner. Doing this will help you relieve anxiety and stress and build trust in your relationship. If your partner is patient with you, listens to you, tries to understand your state of mind, helps you cope with stress, takes ownership of your problems, and genuinely tries to help you through difficult times, you will have found a life partner! However, remember that your partner is not a therapist, so he can't give you **all** the help you need. Instead, let's say it's your partner who suffers from an anxiety disorder; likely, they often feel alone and unloved if they sense a lack of support from you. Some people struggle to express their feelings even to the people they love.

By choosing not to open up to their partners, these people risk damaging their relationship. Since none of us have the power to read the minds of those around us, we can't expect our partners to understand what's bothering us. We need to communicate! Lack of communication alienates us and gives room for misinterpretation. To maintain a healthy relationship with your partner, it is essential to share your feelings and emotions with them.

So far we've seen what anxiety is capable of doing in our relationship if we allow it to creep in and what we can do to combat it. We've said it often, but we'd like to say it again: **the foundation of a solid and lasting relationship must be trust, respect, and communication.** The latter can be difficult to develop within the relationship if we or our partner have an insecure type of attachment. So what can you do to break down the distance between and your partner and foster communication? You can, for example, ask them to go for a walk or have dinner together. A pleasant and safe environment fosters communication.

There are many ways to deal with anxiety in a relationship. We decided to summarize the most important ones in this ten-point list.

1. **TAKE CARE OF YOURSELF.** We can't love others if we don't love ourselves first. Our preoccupied attachment affects our personality. One way to develop self-esteem is to take time for yourself. Love yourself. Take time to do the things you enjoy and take care of your body. A healthy diet and regular physical activity promote proper brain function, relieve stress, relieve anxiety libels, and release serotonin and endorphins, the hormones of happiness!

If you spend time on yourself and feeling good, it will positively affect you, those around you, and your relationship.

2. **SHOW SINCERE INTEREST.** Many people love to be "taken care of" by their better half. If your partner is the type who likes to receive this kind of attention, seek him out and talk to him when you have time. Remember that lack of communication is one of the main causes of misunderstandings in a relationship. Even just a short phone call or message can go a long way. This way you will let your partner know that you are thinking about him at that moment and he will feel loved.

3. **COMMUNICATE.** Communicating is one of the foundations for eliminating anxiety. If you've had a bad day, don't keep your thoughts to yourself; get them out and talk about them with your partner. Of course, you need to be ready to listen when he does the same to you. Talking about whatever is bothering you will help decrease your anxiety levels and relax your mind. Don't give your imagination any room to run wild. Ask questions. Ask your partner how his day was, how he is feeling, take a real interest in him and his feelings and listen carefully. Being able to talk freely with our partners makes us feel understood and loved; we know that we can always rely on someone to take care of us. Even if you don't feel much like talking about it at the time because your day wasn't "great" either, make an effort to talk to each other about it.

4. **BE HONEST.** Would you be happy if your partner lied to you all the time? Would you feel safe in such a relationship? Well, since no one likes to be fooled, don't do that with your partner either. Lies, of any kind, will ruin your relationship! Even a small lie can cause your partner to lose the trust your partner has in you. The building blocks of a healthy and lasting relationship are honesty and openness. If you want to build a stable relationship with your partner, avoid hiding things from them or keeping secrets. There is no such thing as a white lie. Every time you lie or hide things from your partner you are taking away a "building block" from the relationship you have built. Maybe it took you a long time to gain your partner's trust at the beginning of the relationship; so, why ruin it over a lie? The more you share things with your partner, the more trust and love you will get from him/her. Lies only bring with them problems, especially when your partner realizes that you are not sincere. When people start doubting their partners, they start avoiding them, which could eventually lead to a breakup. Think about the consequences of your lies and put yourself in your partner's shoes. Ask yourself: how will your partner feel when they find out the truth? Will he or she still trust me? Will I ever regain his trust? Even one lie can weaken your relationship; it strains and undermines it. It makes your partner insecure about you, insecure about themselves, and all of this creates anxiety, high stress, and communication problems. Is it a lie worth putting up with all this? Be honest.

5. **BE PATIENT.** Patience is a great virtue. Not all of us are patient and meek by nature, so we must strive to cultivate this quality.

When someone does us wrong, the first reaction that this causes in us is anger, frustration, disappointment; even more so if the wrong is done to us by our partner. It is normal to feel this way, but let's not let these feelings take control of our minds. Remember that we also, sometimes unintentionally, hurt others with our words, and when that happens, we want to be forgiven. Let's strive to do the same with others, especially our partners. Maybe your partner didn't mean to hurt you; they simply had a bad day and unloaded the stress on you. Pick a convenient time (when you are calm and the anger has passed), talk to him/her about it and explain how you feel. If you make an effort to be more patient, you will calmly deal with tense and stressful situations. Take the first step!

6. **LAUGH TOGETHER.** Laughter is a natural antidote to stress and tension resulting from anxiety. When we laugh, our blood pressure is lowered, stress is reduced, we stimulate our appetite and set our immune system in motion. Blood pressure is regulated and mood improves! Laughing together with your partner will bring you closer and make it a stronger relationship, and if you've been dealing with some stress during the week, laughing together will help you remember why you love each other. Don't let anxiety take control all the time. Laughing is a great way to relieve tension. How long has it been since you and your partner laughed together? Have fun together and your relationship will be strengthened as a result.

7. **GO ON VACATION TOGETHER.** Stress is one of the main factors that can trigger anxiety symptoms.

One of the best ways to reduce stress is to take your mind off of your daily routine. You and your partner must spend time together.

If you are feeling tired and stressed, why not go on a vacation together, even if it is just for a weekend? Planning a vacation together can help relieve a lot of pressure. Taking a break from the hectic routine and spending time alone will help you communicate, break down the distance between you, and better understand each other. Taking a little break and spending time with your loved one is a healthy and effective way to reduce stress and anxiety caused by an excessive workload.

8. **SPEND TIME WITH YOUR FAMILIES.** The bonds of love and affection become stronger the more your partner knows you and vice versa. Spending time together getting to know each other's families and childhood friends can be a great way to get to know each other better and learn more about the environment our partner grew up in.

9. **SHARE HOBBIES.** Hobbies are a "personal" refuge where everyone seeks joy and peace in times of stress and tries to escape a very anxious period. Some people go to the gym to relieve stress, others like to go for a walk or ride a bike, others like to visit museums, cook, etc. You don't necessarily have to share **all** your hobbies with your partner, but the moment you share **some** of them, you give your partner a chance to get to know you better, understand what you like to do, how you relieve stress and spend time together strengthening your bond.

10. **BE GRATEFUL.** Last on our shortlist, but not least: GRATITUDE. Show your partner how much you care about him, even with small gestures.

Let him know that his support for you is very important. Thank him when he takes the time to listen and be supportive. He will be very happy to know that you appreciate what he does to grow your relationship. Don't be "stingy" with compliments. Showing gratitude to each other, even in the little things, builds respect and trust in your relationship and creates a solid foundation for good communication.

How to Understand the Stages of the Relationship

A couple's relationship is an ongoing process. In the early stages of the relationship, the behaviors and emotions brought into play aim to choose the right person and establish an intimate relationship. In the later stages, however, the emotions aim to maintain a bond with the person chosen as a partner to satisfy the needs for closeness, protection, and support.

But why is it important to understand what stage your relationship is in?

It is important because the quality of a relationship can greatly affect an individual's psychological state. Once you recognize what stage of the relationship you and your partner are going through, you can understand it and each other and thus experience a healthier, more conscious relationship.

Phase 1: Attraction and Courtship

During this phase, unconscious nonverbal strategies are brought into play that is intended to send and receive signals of availability. This is the phase in which you "test the waters" by showing yourself more or less attracted to a person. If the target shows interest, in turn, the signals become more explicit. At the end of this phase, excitement and desire prevail.

In cases where flirting is not aimed at immediate sexual gratification, but the basis is laid for showing a willingness to something more, in addition to attraction and arousal, signals are sought that indicate that the partner is willing to take care of the other, to listen to him, to comfort him, to consider him special.

Phase 2: Falling in Love

The moment the two partners feel they are dealing with the right person, the relationship moves from the attraction phase to the falling in love phase. The initial infatuation is the moment when everything is just beautiful, you feel the "butterflies in your stomach," and you make lots of love. The relationship becomes more intimate, and there is an increase in behaviors that facilitate a sense of mutual well-being. Partners seek physical contact with each other and there is a drastic reduction in anxiety as significant others for the partner are not seen as "a threat".

Numerous studies show that when we fall in love, chemical reactions occur in our brain similar to those triggered by drug use.

The subject of our interest becomes a kind of drug that we need continuously because its presence leads our brain to release a significant amount of hormones such as dopamine, norepinephrine, and phenylethylamine: the same ones activated by drugs. These neurotransmitters act on the pleasure centers and make us feel good. "Unfortunately," this state of physiological hyper-activation lasts from 6 to 9 months.

In this phase we are so caught up in the storm of emotions that we tend to idealize the partner, exalting (often excessively) the positive aspects and similarities and neglecting to take into account the defects and differences in character and behavior. The other person appears perfect in our eyes and we delude ourselves that it will be so forever.

Phase 3: Love

Once the butterflies have flown out, the couple begins to build the foundation of the relationship. This stage is also identified as a "state of happy anxiety" because lovers are in a constant state of worry (their thoughts are always on the other person), but at the same time, they are serene.

This is the stage when:

- One asks questions such as: *"Is she/he the right person for me? Are we going in the same direction, do we want the same things?".* If the answers to the questions are negative, a point is put, while if they are affirmative, the relationship begins to become a real love story;

- The first arguments and confrontations occur. The two lovers no longer see only the positive sides of their partner but begin to truly show themselves for what they are to each other;

- The levels of anxiety and stress grow and become higher and higher because they become aware of all the character sides of the other person and these often turn out to be not perfectly compatible with their personality;

- The frequency of sexual activity decreases;

- The importance of emotional support and the other person's ability to act as a " haven" and as a figure who offers care is increasing. From passion, we move to intimacy, a phase in which the predominant emotions and feelings are of warmth, affection, and trust.

During this phase, the partners become more intimate and discover each other's weaknesses and vulnerabilities resulting in the first differences.

Phase 4: The Post-Romantic Phase

At some point in the relationship, the frequency of sexual exchanges declines further, physical contact decreases, the partners no longer make eye contact with the same frequency and seem to have turned their attention away from each other.

Their energy is directed almost entirely to daily commitments such as children and work.

This phase is called post-romantic because there is enough emotional interdependence between the partners to make their bond solid. There are two dangers in this phase:

- **Neglecting your partner too much.** A relationship always needs to be nurtured. Try to manage your time well. Dedicate time to yourself, your partner, you, and others. Remember that communication is the foundation of your relationship. You must always set aside time for your partner;

- **Boredom.** Being confident in your partner and your relationship decreases anxiety levels, however, there is a risk of experiencing the boredom that comes with habit.

In the post-romantic phase, there can be "crises" in the couple due to unfulfilled expectations. Each of us has different expectations about our relationship. When the reality is different from our expectations, conflicts can arise, and as a result, you may feel a sense of frustration. One of these traps may relate to the frequency of sexuality. In the phase of falling in love, the search for physical closeness leads to a strong sexual attraction, while in more mature phases, hormones such as oxytocin come into play, which dampens sexual desire. This leads to a change in the quality of sexuality, and sex becomes functional to support feelings of closeness and emotional warmth.

Therefore, it is necessary to consciously and objectively observe the progress of your relationship.

In this way, both you and your partner can strive to maintain a balance between the needs for closeness and independence. But how can you assess what stage your love relationship is in?

First, you need to distinguish whether it is a relationship in its infancy or one that has been established over time. If your relationship is just beginning:

1. **Determine if the novelty factor is still alive.** During the early stages of a relationship (attraction and infatuation), there is a strong desire to always be together with the person concerned. Are you finding out his likes, dislikes, hobbies, interests, and ideas? Are you analyzing his personality and habits to determine your degree of compatibility? Do you feel comfortable when you are with him/her?

   Even if you think right now that the person in front of you is perfect, know that he/she is not. Therefore, pay attention to how she/he acts: is she/he affectionate and open? Or is she bossy or grumpy? Does she tend to be unhappy or irritable?

2. **Idealization.** Do you focus only on physical attraction? Chances are when you see the person you're interested in, you blush, your hands shake, and your pulse races.

   If you idealize the person you're dating, think about them often, and can't find any fault with them, then you're still in the infatuation stage.

3. **You want to make a good impression**. Do you always try to behave well and look your best?

   Do you try to please, flatter and woo the person you are dating? During the infatuation phase, you feel more pressure to impress and connect with him/her. The enthusiasm of the moment will encourage you to always do your best and try not to make mistakes. This is why you take more time to prepare for appointments, agree to do activities that usually don't interest you, and give up the company of your friends to spend more time with him/her.

   However, remember that for a relationship to be healthy and long-lasting, you need to be honest and not pretend to be someone else just to impress him/her.

4. **Evaluate**. Are you willing to date her seriously? As you spend more and more time together, you become more comfortable with her and get to know her better. This will help you assess your compatibility more deeply. The person you're dating: does she know how to comfort and support you? Does she trust you and have no problem being honest with you? Does he or she respect your family and friends? Does he or she understand your sense of humor?

5. **Expectations**. As you see each other more often, you will begin to have expectations of each other that may be different and affect your relationship's future. When you consider these deeper aspects, it means that you are moving beyond the infatuation phase and entering the "honeymoon" phase.

If, on the other hand, your relationship with your partner is already underway:

1. **Assess whether you accept your partner's flaws**. If you have reached a realistic stage in the relationship, you will have realized that it is no longer all "sunshine and rainbows" you will have begun to notice aspects that annoy or irritate you. You've become aware that the person in front of you isn't as perfect as they seemed to be in the infatuation phase, but they have their flaws and quirks like you. It is important to understand if you are willing to accept her as she is. If at this stage you can't tolerate your partner's flaws or you think there are aspects you can't improve, you might decide to end the relationship.

2. **Dealing with misunderstandings**. When intimacy is strengthened, disagreements and consequently fights are more likely to arise. Are you willing to compromise and put your partner and your relationship first? If yes, you are going through a phase of the relationship characterized by increased commitment. Loving someone does not mean that there will never be arguments between you. In a relationship, it is normal to have different opinions. The success of your relationship will depend on how you deal with them. If you make communication the basis of your relationship, you will be able to resolve issues peacefully; anxiety and stress will decrease and your relationship will be strengthened. (You will find it helpful to review the communication techniques discussed at the beginning of this chapter.)

3. **Determine the degree of trust.** Can you meet each other's needs? To build a successful relationship, you must trust each other. If instead of making room for feelings like anger and resentment, you cultivate positive emotions and keep calm when your partner talks to you about his or her needs.

In that case, you are definitely in a more mature and fulfilling stage of the relationship. Are you vulnerable with your partner? Can you share your concerns and insecurities with him/her? Can you openly share your feelings with your partner? Do you get angry often? Are you jealous and possessive?

Answering these questions will help you understand the level of trust within your relationship.

4. **Interest in the future**. If you are in a healthy and satisfying relationship, you and your partner will surely talk about plans and dreams for the future. Does your partner have a desire to grow with you? Do you have similar ideas regarding marriage and family? Does he or she envision achieving goals together with you?

5. **A life together.** Are you and your partner planning a life together? You will certainly face challenges together to make it happen. You'll need to put your partner and your relationship first on your list of priorities, and you'll both need to make an effort to develop new habits to meet each other's needs. Maybe you need to make important decisions such as deciding to move in together or buy a house, think about engagement or marriage, and share or combine finances.

In case your relationship is already strong:

1. **Be a team player.** Do you continue to cultivate commitment and loyalty by working together? Even if you've known each other for a long time and are comfortable with each other, a relationship requires ongoing work and commitment from both partners.

    Your relationship is a mature one, so you need to rely on each other, fulfill or keep your promises, be comfortable with your responsibilities and roles, and make your partner your anchor in difficult times.

2. **Watch out for boredom.** When the relationship is stable, romance fades more and more. In this case, it may seem difficult to know what stage of the relationship you are in. Examine whether the habits shared with your partner. Are you feeling bored or frustrated? If so, carve out time to do something fun together, open yourself up to new activities, or try something you enjoyed doing as a kid.

3. **Anticipate your partner's wants and needs.** At this stage, you and your partner already know each other very well and can anticipate each other's needs in difficult times and everyday life. Knowing and giving importance to your partner's needs before he even makes requests allows you to take care of her every day. For example, if you know that he/she had a bad day, you can do something nice for him/her or encourage him/her to take some time for himself/herself to practice some hobbies or go out with friends.

If you are not sure what your partner's wants and needs are, talk to him/her about it. Try to figure out if there is a problem in your relationship if he needs more attention or some recreation. Listen carefully and try to understand what his needs are without interrupting while he is talking and without getting defensive.

4. **Reserve time to spend together.** Carving out time each day to communicate with your partner is very important to strengthen your bond. If you both have children and/or work, it can be difficult to maintain a healthy, stable, and loving relationship due to numerous commitments and stresses. Do you do several activities at once? Do you spend more time on your children or work and neglect your partner? If so, your relationship may suffer. If you and your partner find yourself in this situation, try this:

   - Express appreciation and gratitude. You could thank him for something he does, such as making coffee or dinner. Let him know that you appreciate what he does.

   - Express affection. You've known your partner for a long time, so you know what she likes; surprise her! No big things are needed. Give her a hug when she's not expecting it, say *"I love you,"* write her a card or give her a flower.

5. **Communicate**. Take 20 minutes a day to tell each other what you did during the day. Listening to each other helps relieve anxiety, tension, and stress and unplug together.

(You may find it helpful to review the chapter on communication and active listening in this regard).

6. **Mutual Respect.** Respect is one of the fundamental pillars of having a successful relationship. If you always treat each other with love, even when you have differences of opinion, you will be able to base your relationship on commitment and strength.

   You will put aside the expectations you have of your partner and you will be able to accept your partner for both their good and bad points. If you are unable to cultivate respect in your relationship, consider embarking on a course of couples therapy.

If mutual respect is lacking to the point that either partner becomes physically or verbally violent, seek help from a psychologist. Violence should not be accepted at any stage of a relationship.

Unfortunately, sometimes, despite the commitment and goodwill, some relationships become toxic for one or both of them. There are many reasons why a relationship ends, and almost all of them stem from a lack of trust and mutual respect. How can you deal with the end of a relationship?

When to End a Relationship

If you and your partner are not practicing mindfulness, you may feel the need to impose your personal beliefs on the relationship. You must be willing to compromise and find a middle ground.

If you realize that your partner is not willing to meet you halfway, you may decide that ending the relationship is the best course of action. However, in this case, you need to be objective about your relationship and you need to make a decision.

Ask yourself: *is my partner showing that he or she is not willing to build a stable relationship? Does he run away from difficulties instead of being willing to face them together?*

Does he always want to impose his point of view without finding a compromise between how I see the situation and how he sees it? Do you feel loved and cared for? Does your partner help you through difficult times? Does he/she support you when you face difficult times and feel sad and upset? Does your partner encourage you to pursue your dreams?

At this point, think back to the list you wrote at the beginning of the chapter about what you look for in your ideal partner. Examining your relationship critically will help you see where your relationship stands and make a decision, it will help you see if working together with your partner on your issues will get you through this time of crisis or if the current situation is not worth your time and energy and that it is time to move on.

Since committing to a relationship is like flying a plane, you should ask yourself if you are also supportive of your partner. Ask yourself: *Am I present and cooperative? When my partner is struggling, am I ready to help and support them? Do I put our relationship first? Or am I always too busy and not giving him/her enough time?*

A successful relationship requires both partners to work together to make it successful. Your commitment alone is not enough to save the relationship if your partner is not emotionally available to you. But how can you tell if your relationship is worth your time and energy or if it's time to put an end to it? Here's what you can do:

- **REFLECT ON YOUR PROBLEMS.**

Ask yourself: *Are the problems that got us to this point fixable?*

In most cases, relationship problems can be resolved with commitment from both of you, but when one of you is unwilling to give in or do your part, it means that the relationship is out of balance and you are no longer able to commit to compromise: it's probably time to put an end to it.

- **ENVISION YOUR FUTURE.**

Ask yourself: *Do I see myself next to this person in the future?*

Imagining the future together is essential in a lasting relationship. If looking ahead you can't imagine yourself next to your partner and even think you'll be better off a different person, then it's most likely time to end the relationship.

- **RANCHES.**

Sometimes problems can arise in a relationship that causes deep emotional wounds (such as cheating), and when this happens, you are overwhelmed with negative thoughts. Perhaps you have decided to forgive your partner but, despite this, you always think the worst and you can no longer create within your relationship the trust needed to move forward. If you have realized that this pain leads you to be always suspicious and extremely jealous of your partner to the point that your relationship is "hell" due to the continuous lack of trust, perhaps leaving is the most appropriate choice.

- **ALWAYS FIGHTING.**

You may have happened to think: *"All we do now is fight!"*

Frequent arguments, even over trifles, are one of the main signs that reveal when the relationship is in danger. It is normal in a relationship to argue occasionally, but in a relationship that works, these occasions of conflict are an opportunity for both partners to get to know each other better, feel close and learn how to better manage the relationship. In a healthy relationship, disagreements help strengthen the relationship between the partners even more.

While arguing itself can be a positive action within a healthy relationship, repeated and unnecessary bickering often does not indicate that love is ending instead.

Think: do you and your partner fight all the time?

Do you have negative feelings about each other? Is every occasion useful to express anger, disappointment and to accuse your partner of all his mistakes in the present and the past?

If you experience brief moments of happiness following a social event, a vacation, or a sexual relationship, but most of your days are made up of constant conflict, it means that the relationship is beginning to degenerate. Remember that constant conflict drives you away from each other. At this point you have two options:

1. come together: work together on communication, listening, empathy, and all the aspects we have analyzed in this chapter;

2. end your relationship: if neither of you changes your position, if neither of you makes a step forward towards the other, then it means that probably the fight is just one of the ways to avoid the end of the relationship.

To have a lasting and successful relationship, you both need to work on your relationship and strive to meet each other's needs. If you are not going to do this, why keep fighting?

- **IRRECONCILABLE DIFFERENCES.**

You may have said to your partner: *"What happened to you? I don't recognize you anymore!"*

Perhaps as you continue with your relationship, you will have realized that your partner has characteristics that you didn't realize while dating; perhaps you have discovered that he has a very different type of upbringing than you or you have different values; perhaps he has changed some of his ways, or perhaps he no longer has enough time for you because he is taken up with other occupations and friends.

In the "falling in love" phase, you feel so calm and happy that you see only the beautiful and positive things about the person in front of you. When the "falling in love" phase ends, it is normal to start seeing all the flaws in your partner, and this leads you to see with other eyes the person you once loved deeply or thought you loved. You begin, thus, to see things clearly and, unfortunately, you realize that there is no love. As time goes by, everything that you used to like and could tolerate, you now no longer tolerate.

This can cause some confusion in your partner, who does not change his habits since you had never complained before.

Another major reason why you start to create a gap between partners is the lack of time. Usually, women are more willing to devote time, availability, and involvement to their relationship, while men are a bit more reluctant to give it. If you and your partner don't devote enough time to your relationship, if you don't compromise to meet each other's needs, and if you don't communicate, your relationship won't survive for long.

- **EMOTIONAL DISTANCE.**

You may have found yourself thinking: *"I feel my partner is distant like he's not there anymore."*

You may come to think this when you try to connect with your partner, but he is distant, you try to chat with him, but he is distant. When you and your partner interrupt any form of communication (verbal, sexual, emotional), your relationship suffers a kind of "blackout" perceived precisely as emotional distance. It is as if you unconsciously decide to limit all contact with your partner; emotions are inhibited and energies and resources are used elsewhere. A deep emotional distance indicates, first of all, a lack of communication in the couple. Also, it indicates that, instead of consulting each other to create a common reality that meets the needs of both, the partners make decisions on their own, based on their values and without taking into account the needs of the other.

- **BOREDOM.**

Ask yourself: *"Am I bored with my partner? Are all the days the same?"*

If you wake up every morning depressed and out of sorts, the vitality in your relationship may be gone. Of course, we can't wake up euphoric all the time; everyone's life is full of boring moments, and even those who live happily ever after sometimes wake up bored, out of energy, and apathetic as if something interesting, exciting, or fascinating could never happen to them again.

Usually, when you feel bored and frustrated (but not dissatisfied with your relationship) your partner acts as a refuge to all these unpleasant feelings.

You cannot attribute boredom solely to the relationship. Evaluate all of the external situations that might extinguish enthusiasm throughout the day. Sometimes people think that a relationship goes on automatically, when in fact it needs a lot of work and willpower. A relationship begins to deteriorate when even one of the two no longer shows interest. If regardless of the cause of the estrangement, your relationship is no longer a resource you can count on, and the feelings that accompany this slow end to the relationship are distractions and a lack of purpose and motivation, you might broach the subject with your partner and at that point decide **together** whether to work on your relationship by committing to come together by nurturing your relationship, or to move away for good.

- **LIFE CHANGES.**

If your partner has recently changed jobs, his or her routine has likely changed and he or she has begun to take time away from your relationship; you may have thought, *"Since he or she started that new job, he or she doesn't pay attention to me anymore. It's like I don't exist for him/her anymore."*

Changes (whether it's work, home, or country) are never easy, but with mutual support, everything can be addressed and overcome.

However, sometimes (especially in teenagers), a change can bring out the fact that the foundation of your relationship is no longer solid and that it was only situations that kept you together: for example living in a certain house, in a particular city, or because there were certain conditions. Change generates a lot of stress and anxiety within a relationship, but at the same time, it can shed light on what is no longer going as it should. Dealing with these situations can make you realize if it is possible to put a positive spin on your relationship and come out of it better and stronger, or if it is time to end it because it is a long-dead relationship.

- **BETRAYAL.**

When one of the partners gets to the point of cheating on the other, it means that something in the relationship is wrong. Sex is one of the most important bonds in a relationship. Cheating on your partner means taking away from your relationship one of the elements that make it unique and exclusive.

When there are multiple betrayals within a relationship, it means that the relationship is no longer intimate but is just an arrangement of convenience and only lasts as long as both of you hold up the game. Creating a moment of intimacy in a situation like this is almost impossible since the emotional territory has already been repeatedly violated. This is one of the situations where it's time to end the relationship.

- **LACK OF TRUST.**

In this chapter, we have talked a lot about the importance of trust, how to create it, how to increase it, and how to regain it, but we have also seen that the latter is not always possible. In addition to being one of the cornerstones of love, trusting your partner avoids clashes and arguments dictated by blind jealousy. If your relationship is full of lies, mistrust, jealousy, and infidelity, the relationship will likely destabilize and the first quarrels will begin to surface. All these problems, moreover, can lead you to suffer more than you should.

When you begin to feel the uncontrollable urge to keep an eye on your partner, trying to understand who he sees during the day in your absence or with whom he writes on various social networks even though he has given you no reason to doubt him, then it may be that trust is lacking within the couple. In this case, you should work on yourself and eliminate the negative thoughts as we have already seen at the beginning of the chapter. You should also understand where your insecurity comes from and do this with self-awareness and a professional's help. If not "treated", jealousy can wear down your relationship and your partner may eventually decide to end your relationship.

Thinking about ending a relationship and doing it are two very different things. Sometimes we plan for the end of a relationship, trying to find the best way to make this decision easy or we freeze for fear of hurting the other person.

It is important to be able to open our eyes to reality by acting like adults and identifying the signs that indicate the end of a relationship. Relationships are an important part of our lives and everyone has had to end one. Identifying when it is over or needs to end can be crucial to your physical and mental health. But how can you be sure that a relationship no longer has a future?

The tips in this chapter can help you strengthen or recover your relationship and make it stronger. If, however, reflecting on these issues has made you realize there are problems, stop for a moment. When deciding such importance, you need to be clear-headed. Don't decide to end the relationship in a moment of impulsiveness, instability, or at the end of a hell of a week (you'll end up blaming the relationship for all your problems).

How to Deal with Ending a Relationship

Deciding to end a relationship is never easy. Even if you practice self-awareness, breakups can be extremely painful. Sometimes people can't handle the separation and end up getting back together. If, however, you and your partner don't make the proper changes, you may find yourself in a more unpleasant situation than before.

Most of the time, after enough time has passed, you'll both be right back where you started and will most likely separate again or stay together even if your relationship makes you unhappy.

Although separating can be difficult and distressing, remember the reasons why you decided to end your relationship.

If you made this decision, it's because you carefully assessed the situation and realized that your partner was failing to meet your needs. Thinking about all the reasons that led you to make this difficult choice will help you get through the pain of the moment. When you decide to put an end to it, this does not automatically end your feelings for the person with whom you shared a lot of time, sometimes even years. However, going back to such a person will not make you happy. In the long run, it will be healthier for you to move on, heal from your breakup and find someone who can give you what you need.

Even if the relationship has become toxic and damaging, people don't always choose to leave their partners. This is because knowing your partner well gives an illusory "stability" to the relationship, a sense of safety and security. They know exactly how to react and how their partner will react, and what to expect from their partners and themselves even if they find themselves in a cyclone of physical and/or psychological abuse. Even if their partner's behavior causes pain and humiliation, they are willing to accept it as long as they remain in their "comfort zone" because the predictability of the relationship and their partner's reactions instills a sense of security. Very often people with low self-esteem and anxiety disorders choose to surround themselves with people who reinforce their perception that they are unworthy of being loved. This causes people with low self-esteem to become trapped in toxic relationships instead of seeking out loving and caring partners.

To break out of this vicious cycle, sufferers of this disorder must seek professional foreign support.

Through therapy, appropriate medication and a great deal of introspection will be able to change themselves, abandon toxic relationships of which they are victims, and develop new healthy relationships. To change, however, you must **recognize** and **accept** the need for change; only then will you be able to cut ties with the toxic people in your life and give more space to new relationships that will help you progress in your change.

We have already seen when it is time to end a relationship; in this subchapter, you will see how **to be consistent** with your decision. Those who have an insecure attachment style may be so frightened by the idea of leaving a person that they lose sight of rationality. If you have this attachment style, stop and think carefully and weigh the pros and cons; this way you can realize that ending a relationship with a person with whom you can no longer be yourself will be a real liberation, which could pave the way to happiness.

If you've realized that your relationship is toxic and unhealthy and you've decided to end it, you should implement a strategy that will help you be consistent with the decision you've made without retracing your steps, only to be hurt again and experience further anxiety and pain. Here are 10 tips that will help you during this process:

1. **PROCESS THE LOSS.** In the face of any loss, it is important to process the separation.

Even in the case of the end of a love affair is very often spoken of grief processing (in this case in the sense of loss) because the abandonment and finding themselves alone, brings with it much pain and suffering. In these cases, as in mourning, it may happen to go through 5 stages of processing: denial, anger, negotiation, depression, and acceptance. Therefore, it is important to live these emotions and perhaps even share them with a friend or a specialist.

2. **RELY ON YOUR SUPPORT SYSTEM.** Breakups are always painful and eventually, you will need someone to rely on and share your feelings with. Share your emotions and feelings with the people who love you; spending more time with your family and friends will help you get through this. When you lose an important person in your life, it's natural to feel unhappy and alone. Don't suppress your feelings. Cry when you feel the need to; it will help you get through the pain of the end of your relationship.

3. **BECOME AWARE OF WHAT HAPPENED.** Take your time to analyze and understand what happened in your relationship and why it ended. Try to remember what made you fall in love and then what caused those feelings to die out. Don't blame anyone for the end of the relationship but just try to understand the dynamics, responsibilities, and factors that made this story start and then end. Don't think of yourself as the victim or the perpetrator, but try to have an objective look at what happened so that you can learn from your mistakes.

4. **DON'T USE OTHER PEOPLE AS A REPLACEMENT.** It's okay to vent, but don't use the people close to you (children, friends, or new acquaintances) as a weapon against the ex or as a replacement for not feeling alone. Try to be honest with those around you and remember that those around you may be a good shoulder to cry on but may not be able to give you all the help you need.

5. **RESPECT YOURSELF AND THE PRIVACY OF OTHERS.** After separation, you may feel a little lost, as if a part of you has disappeared somewhere. Resist the temptation to search and stalk your ex on social media and avoid publicizing the breakup as an outlet. It's never a good idea.

6. **RECOVER YOUR SELF-ESTEEM.** When faced with a breakup or the end of a relationship, the first feeling is to lose your self-esteem. Thus, it can be useful to try to become aware of what happened and understand that not everything depended on you. Practice self-awareness and increase your self-esteem (you can find many great tips at the beginning of the chapter).

7. **BE PREPARED FOR THE URGE TO GET BACK TOGETHER.** As you go through all of this, there is a chance that at some point, you will think about getting back together with your ex. You will almost exclusively remember the good things about your relationship without thinking about the hard times and all the reasons why you decided to leave him. Before you get in touch with your ex or answer his or her calls, think about the difficult times you had with him/her. The feelings of sadness and loneliness might become so overwhelming that they push you to look for him/her again, but this does not mean that you are a weak person.

Sometimes, it is easier to go back to old relationships than to start new ones. Seek help and advice from your closest friends and family members. If you decide to give your ex another try, don't blame yourself; if you conclude once again that ending the relationship was the right decision, remember that you will be able to move on with a little time.

8. **LET GO AND MOVE ON**. Closing with the past is one of the decisive steps to overcome the end of a relationship. It is one of the longest and most complicated steps, but little by little, it is necessary to overcome it. If jealousy or remorse assail you, try to distract yourself.

9. **CHOOSE HEALTHY WAYS TO DEAL WITH STRESS AND SADNESS.** When you're going through tough times, it can be easy to adopt unhealthy habits. Make an effort to take care of yourself.

   - Play sports. Physical activity produces serotonin, which is a hormone that helps reduce anxiety and stress and gives you a sense of well-being. Also, dedicating some time to your body and taking care of yourself can make you feel better in general.

   - Strive for proper nutrition.

   - Rediscover your old hobbies and keep busy with your favorite activities.

   - Listen to relaxing music

   - Watch your favorite movies or programs

- Take care of yourself, for example, by taking long baths.

- Take walks.

- Get enough sleep.

These activities will make you feel better and ensure that your mental and physical health is not compromised after the breakup.

10. **VOLUNTEER.** Taking an interest in others will take your mind off your problems, give your life meaning and help you not feel lonely. Helping others helps you feel valuable and connected to other people.

Accepting the end of a love affair is the turning point for moving past the closure of the story. Loving yourself and learning to take care of yourself is the best way to start putting yourself out there again. Don't rush into a new relationship right away so you don't feel alone. Take the time to process what happened and learn from your mistakes. This will help you regain respect and love for yourself and others.

Conclusion

We hope that this book has provided you with the help you need to make the necessary changes to your relationship so that you can make it stronger. By making small changes, starting with yourself, you will be able to deal with everyday anxiety and worries and build a healthy, happy relationship. Love, respect, compassion, understanding, and empathy are the keys to a successful relationship that stands the test of time.

The information provided in this book is not intended to replace the help you can get from a professional. If you or your partner suffers from an anxiety disorder, we recommend that you get expert help. If you find that this book's guidance is not enough or you need help applying its concepts, consider couples therapy.